NATURE *and*
HUMAN PERSONALITY

Homoeopathic Archetypes

NATURE *and* HUMAN PERSONALITY

Homoeopathic Archetypes

Catherine R. Coulter

With Foreword by
Stephanie K. Stevens, M.D., M.P.H.

Ninth House Publishing

BERKELEY SPRINGS, WEST VIRGINIA
2002

This book is, in part, an abridgment by Catherine R. Coulter
of selected chapters from her previously published works,
Portraits of Homoeopathic Medicines:
Psychophysical Analyses of Selected Constitutional Types,
Volumes 1, 2, and 3.
These books are available from
Ninth House Publishing.

EDITOR Suzanne Wakefield
COVER DESIGN Diane Beasley
ILLUSTRATIONS AND COVER ILLUSTRATION Alex Coulter

Printed in the United States of America
by McNaughton & Gunn

Published by Ninth House Publishing
33 Fairfax Street, Berkeley Springs, West Virginia 25411
Telephone: 1-800-336-1695 • Web Site: www.homeopathyworks.com

LIBRARY OF CONGRESS CATALOGING-IN-PUBLICATION DATA

Coulter, Catherine R.
  Nature and human personality : homoeopathic archetypes /
Catherine R. Coulter ; with foreword by Stephanie K. Stevens.
    p.   cm.
  Includes bibliographical references and index.
  ISBN 0-9713082-4-1
  1. Homeopathy—Materia medica and therapeutics.
  2. Typology. 3. Medicine. 4. Psychology.
RX631.C68   2000
615.5'32—dc21   00-033314

Aude Sapere
(Venture to Try)

EPIGRAPH TO SAMUEL HAHNEMANN'S
Organon of Medicine

Acknowledgments

I would like to extend special thanks to my editor, Suzanne Wakefield, for her friendly assistance and expert advice—also to Marian Coulter for her valuable comments on the text.

Contents

Foreword

My fascination with homoeopathy began many years ago when I came across Boericke's *Materia Medica With Repertory* in a yard sale one leisurely Sunday morning. Although I had no knowledge of homoeopathy at that time in my life, I was intrigued by the contents of this standard reference text. As the years passed, and I shifted my career focus from public health policy to medicine, Boericke's *Materia Medica* maintained a special place in my library, first at home and then in my office at the hospital. I did not understand the information that it contained, nor did I have any concept of how the information could possibly be applicable to treating my patients. After all, I was a physician, conventionally trained in the science of modern, scientific medicine. However, despite the fact that my medical colleagues would view the homoeopathic *Materia Medica* as a product of now inferior and outdated medical theories, the text held me captive to its mysteries.

My personal and professional evolution to embrace a holistic approach to health and wellness was born out of my public health roots, in which health promotion and disease prevention are valued rather than illness care and management, which is the focus of modern allopathic medicine. What followed was a personal and career transition away from conventional medicine into the fascinating realm of holistic health practice and homoeopathy.

As the old adage goes, "When the student is ready, the teacher will appear." And so it was for me and my study of homoeopathy, under the tutelage of Catherine R. Coulter, a modern-day homoeopathic master and teacher. As a conventionally trained physician of Western medicine, I was amazed at the power of these ultradiluted remedies (which, when chemically analyzed, contain only the milk sugar that serves as the vehicle for holding the remedy) to cure con-

ditions and diseases for which there were no cures in modern conventional medicine. How was this possible? What was the mecha-
nism of action? Why was the medical community so resistant to this
form of alternative medicine? These are just some of the many questions that need to be answered. The answers will be provided when
the science of quantum physics is applied toward the understanding
of the human energy field, and when it elucidates the energetics
that underlie many of the alternative and complementary disciplines,
such as homoeopathy.

Catherine R. Coulter's three-volume *Portraits of Homoeopathic
Medicines: Psychophysical Analyses of Selected Constitutional Types,*
and the chapters in this book, which are her abridgments of that earlier work, are like no other homoeopathic texts. Her organization of
the material, focusing on the major constitutional archetypes, coupled with her eloquent narrative style, which includes well-known
literary and historic characters, brings the homoeopathic constitutional remedies to life.

Like all holistic health disciplines, homoeopathic remedies work
to correct imbalances that result in *dis*-ease by strengthening the individual's life force and restoring harmony and balance to the organism at all levels—mind, body, and spirit. As the medical community
in the United States grows in its acceptance of medical pluralism and
catches up with the rest of the world (homoeopathy is the second
most popular form of health care in the world, according to a 1993
report from the World Health Organization), homoeopathy will regain its place in this country as a major health care alternative.

Stephanie K. Stevens, M.D., M.P.H.

Introduction

When Samuel Hahnemann founded his new medical discipline, homoeopathy, in 1796, he not only founded a new method of prescribing drugs to heal the sick; he also discovered a whole new way of viewing the world we live in and of understanding human nature. Every substance on this planet (he maintained), whether vegetable, animal, or mineral, contains locked within itself curative powers. This particular energy has only to be released for living or inert matter to become a potent healing agent. The crucial question that poses itself is, how does one identify the particular healing powers in nature?

Samuel Hahnemann (1755-1843) was born in Meissen, Saxony, the gifted son of poor but educated parents (his father was a painter of porcelain in the porcelain works for which Meissen is famous). After completing his education, he started on a career as a physician, but became progressively more disillusioned with what he learned. Finally, he renounced medicine altogether and for some years made a living by translating chemistry books and medical texts. It was while translating a book on Peruvian bark (quinine) that Hahnemann made a discovery that was to redirect his life. Dissatisfied with the traditional explanation of how quinine acts to cure malaria, he decided to try the substance on himself and observe its effects. What materialized was that he developed the symptoms of malaria—chills, drowsiness, heart palpitations, trembling, prostration through all the limbs, rigidity of the joints—and this discovery, acting as a catalyst to his medical thinking, gave birth to the science of homoeopathy.

If quinine, which causes the symptoms of malaria in a healthy person, could *cure* malaria in an ill one, this signified that it acts as a "similar" medicine—curing the disease by virtue of its ability to produce the same symptoms in the healthy. After repeating the same experiment with several other plant substances and experiencing the same results, Hahnemann generalized this observation into the "Law of Similars" and formulated the fundamental principle of the homoeopathic doctrine, *similia similibus curentur* (let likes be cured by likes); hence the name "homoeopathy," from the Greek *homoios pathos,* meaning "similar disease."

Hahnemann had next to devise a systematic method for ascertaining the actual curative powers of various substances found in nature, in order to use them as similars. This is where his genius came particularly to the fore. He discovered and elaborated a method known as the "proving" (from the German *Pruefung,* meaning "test" or "trial") by which minute doses of a substance are administered on a systematic basis to healthy persons over a period of days or weeks, and the symptoms elicited thereby are recorded. This procedure revealed that every substance displayed a set of symptoms peculiar to itself, so that the "similarity" could be established by matching the clinically "proven" symptoms to a patient's complex of symptoms. In this way, by treating not the disease per se but rather a patient's idiosyncratic set of symptoms, homoeopathy *individualizes* every case. Furthermore, since the provings elicited mental symptoms as well as physical ones, homoeopathy denies any qualitative distinction or artificial separation between physical, emotional, and mental symptoms—assuming that all processes within the organism are interdependent. Any attempt at treating an organ or part of the body must be treatment of the whole body, the whole patient. Physical illnesses have a mental aspect, while mental illnesses have a physical aspect, and the prescription of drugs must be based on a consideration of both categories of symptoms as viewed in their dynamic interaction.

This "holistic" approach, a method of addressing a medicine to the totality of a person's symptoms, is called "constitutional prescribing"; and the expression "constitutional remedy" signifies the medicinal substance that encompasses the sum total of an individual's personality picture—as manifested in his looks, manner, voice, speech, gestures, responses, thoughts, feelings, fears, hopes, tastes, strengths and weaknesses, disposition and temperament (both in illness and in health)—as well as his common or idiosyncratic physical symptoms. A person is said to be a *Phosphorus*, a *Pulsatilla*, a *Silica*, or some other "constitutional type" according to the "proven" natural substance that his totality of symptoms most closely approximates.

Another word that periodically crops up in any treatise on homeopathy is "potentization." This refers to the method of preparing the remedies. During the process of his provings, Hahnemann stumbled on a significant paradox: the more diluted a medicinal substance, the longer and stronger was its curative action. Every successive dilution (prepared according to a specified procedure of succussing the liquids and triturating the solids) releases increasingly *more* of its innate healing energy. Thus the remedies, in their different strengths or dilutions, are alluded to as "potencies."

Restricted as these archetypal pictures are by considerations of space, they tend to be selective rather than comprehensive. In every picture certain features are emphasized, certain themes developed, and certain nuances brought to the fore because they appear quintessential to the type. To illustrate these points, examples have been taken from history and literature. Historic and literary figures portray human characteristics in concentrated (or archetypal) form; and because they have become familiar parts of our cultural heritage, any allusion to them suggests to the reader a host of associations that bring the remedy's specific personality into clear focus.

It is important to bear in mind that the characteristics of the different constitutional types can, and to a certain extent do, overlap. In real life the typological boundaries are fluid, and there are no absolutes. A *Sepia* can sparkle with cheerfulness and mirth, a *Lycopodium* can be truly unassuming, and an *Arsenicum album* can be quite unconcerned with his health. In choosing to emphasize specific traits of a personality type one necessarily simplifies a complex nature that displays features of other remedy types as well. Also, few individuals are covered by a single remedy throughout their lifetime.

The stresses and strains of physical or emotional trauma, job or vocation, marriage and family life—or the lack of same—all leave their imprint and promote changes and modifications in an individual, who will gravitate around several constitutional types. But when prescribing for a patient, generally one constitutional picture will predominate at any given moment.

Note that the charts at the end of the chapters, cursory as they are, serve as a reminder that the homoeopathic emphasis on character analysis and human typology is not an end in itself, but a means of establishing the most "similar" remedy for purposes of healing in both common ailments and the more serious diseases.

The time is at hand for the homoeopathic archetypes to become a part of our general culture—for the *Sulphur, Lachesis,* and *Natrum muriaticum* personality types to be recognized by individuals concerned with their physical and emotional well-being, as well as by healers who wish to use homoeopathy in conjunction with their particular discipline. The following twelve time-honored and time-proven remedies have been selected as the ones that those who practice homoeopathy most consistently turn to for assistance in illness and empowerment in health.

Catherine R. Coulter

Phosphorus

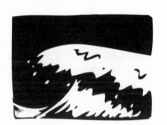

The homoeopathic remedy is made from the luminescent element phosphorus, the only nonradioactive substance capable of producing its own light. The name originates from the Greek word *phos,* meaning "light," and a form of *phoros,* meaning "bringer"—hence "bringer of light." Both the etymology and the associations evoked by the element provide fitting keys to the *Phosphorus* personality.

Anyone who has been by the ocean at night has seen the flecks of phosphorus dancing in the foam or gleaming in the swells. This sparkling element captures the attention, and the *Phosphorus* individual has a similar eye-catching appeal; he attracts by his looks and manner. Particularly arresting are the eyes: shining with a soft, luminous quality that draws another closer or with a captivating brightness, they are emblematic of the whole person. No other constitutional type is emotionally more responsive to another's wavelength or more intuitive in dealing with people. All of his impulses and mannerisms reveal a readiness to establish warm communication with his fellow human beings. He predisposes others toward himself by little verbal kindnesses, warm praise, or touching consideration—

and at times by almost undue generosity, giving up for a friend more than anyone else would think reasonable.*

Occasionally, the *Phosphorus* individual will possess a quiet, refined personality that emits a gentle luminescence. He is friendly, sympathetic, and clearly likes people, but is somewhat shy and reserved. More often he is lively. Just as the element generates light spontaneously, so this bright, bubbling individual throws off sparks from a seemingly inexhaustible internal source of light. In either case, the type is made for happiness. He knows how to enjoy himself and is easily entertained; he also knows how to entertain others. He is a good conversationalist—imaginative, seldom tedious or overbearing, often bringing an artistic flair to the mundane. He is quick to see the humorous side of things and is ever ready to laugh, even at himself, fully appreciating the attention. Rather than being critical of humanity, he is diverted by its follies, inconsistencies, and weaknesses and tries to ignore the unpleasant aspects of life.

The *Phosphorus* allure is in part sparkle, in part a genuine desire to make others happy—and he will work hard to these ends. He is an attentive and highly reactive listener, entering wholeheartedly into another's good fortune and empathizing fully with his hardships: "Yes, I know *just* how you feel. You had no choice but to act as you did. The same thing happened to me when . . ." And, leaning forward in the chair to get as near to his interlocutor as possible, or placing a soothing hand on his arm to physically demonstrate his sympathy, he contributes some perceptive remark that illuminates the other's concerns. In comforting others, *Phosphorus* instinctively finds the right words, tone of voice, and gestures. For this reason, together with his talent for making others feel good in and about themselves, this type often enjoys considerable healing abilities in a

---

*N.B.: For stylistic purposes and to avoid cumbersome phraseology, the masculine gender has been employed throughout this book to denote both sexes, except when characteristics relate more particularly to the female.

professional capacity. A *Phosphorus* doctor or nurse has only to enter the room and throw out an encouraging word, or lay his or her hands on a sufferer, to make him feel better.

Phosphorus also makes it his credo to be kind. If a hostess asks him what he thinks of her homemade coconut cake, even if he dislikes coconut he will say, with engaging frankness and utter conviction, "It was *the* most delicious cake I've eaten in months. How *did* you make it?" And with his expansive impulses he extends kindness and warmth even to newly formed or chance acquaintances—persons in whom he has intrinsically little interest, apart from his generally amicable nature.

Whenever the exigencies of his studies and numerous friends permitted, one *Phosphorus* college student would donate a day visiting detention homes and reformatories for juvenile delinquents. There he instructed them in whatever skill took their fancy—carpentry, playing the saxophone or guitar, sketching, yoga, soccer, or basketball. The inmates had just to mention their interest and this master of innumerable skills cheerfully undertook to teach them. "Not that I expect to reform a single soul," he remarked. "But they seem to look forward to my visits—and some are great kids! Also, I feel that I should give them some of the chances in life that I had." Of course, that which he could not give others was his *Phosphorus* amiability, compassion, and generous impulses.

On the conscious level, this sympathetic person is sincerely caring and solicitous. On another level, however, by ingratiating himself he is securing, in return, the love and special attention to which *he* feels entitled. For his sparkle proceeds also from a self-love. He considers himself more intuitive, more gifted, more sensitive and refined, more generous and helpful than the ordinary mortal ("It's amazing how much I do for others!"). He can be quite fascinated with his person—not merely vain about his looks, but more significantly, viewing himself as a latter-day Prometheus whose talents, like the fire stolen from heaven, enrich mankind. One individual may say, "I have a very special way with children. I can charm them into performing better than any other teacher"; another will volunteer, "I am talented in any art form I choose, but I am most gifted in . . ."; a third describes himself as "as easy and pleasant a person to get along with as you will ever encounter." And then he may append, "For fifty years I've kept my wife happy and our marriage a success. Now *that's* an accomplishment!" And it is! But in so saying, *Phosphorus* may overlook the fact that a substantial portion of the credit might belong to another. Yet the type's captivating manner and patently good intentions permit him to say and do things that in another person would be considered conceited or in poor taste. So motivated by generous impulses is he, so abundant in charm, that notwithstanding his egotism, he manages to win others' affectionate approval.

In the person with a strong urge to entertain, please, and draw attention to himself, one method is self-dramatization. Indeed, *Phosphorus* is able to infuse drama and romance into a chance encounter with an old school friend. He can magnify into a near-disaster such an everyday occurrence as milk boiling over on the stove. The more momentous events in his life become endowed with a cosmic significance in which all must share. Either he is confronting some new crisis or he is merely a stone's throw away from becoming a celebrity; either he is on the verge of certain financial ruin or he is launching a world-staggering scheme that is going to reap him millions!

There is an undeniable "prima donna" aspect to this constitutional type; he is the sun around whom the rest of humanity revolves. But he is a generous, benign prima donna who, in his own enjoyment of it, wishes to include others in his life drama. He does not so much pull others into his orbit (there is no coercion; they are free to leave anytime they so desire) as he offers them a chance to participate in the merriment and excitement. The drawback is that a *Phosphorus* of "star" mentality might promise more than he can deliver. Try as he might, he cannot always infect others with his own sense of drama and joie de vivre.

Like the flecks of phosphorus that glimmer and swirl with every impulse of the sea, the human *Phosphorus* is responsive to the subtlest influences of his environment. This individual can be overly sensitive to odors, sounds, sunlight or artificial light, and especially to changes in temperature or barometric pressure. The nervous, easily excited disposition is likewise susceptible to various fears: of the dark, of illness, of impending misfortune; and sometimes the fears are free floating and undefined. One fear peculiar to this type is that of thunderstorms. He cringes from the flashes of lightning and trembles at the sound of thunder. It is as if he were already generating enough of his own electricity, and more throws him off-balance.

All his fears and anxieties are exaggerated by solitude—and ameliorated by company. The gregarious *Phosphorus* soul not only needs people around to feel whole, he might even need actual physical contact. He himself is demonstratively affectionate, liking to kiss and hug and touch, and seems always to be seeking reassurance from the presence, palpably felt, of others.

Furthermore, so responsive is he to his human brothers that he cannot be truly happy unless those around him are happy also. This is another reason for his efforts to ingratiate himself. Disagreeable impressions or unpleasant feelings make him physically ill, bringing on trembling, head or stomach pains, insomnia, or palpitations. For that matter, even pleasurable emotions can affect him similarly. He begins quivering or is kept awake at night by the excitement of a stimulating conversation, a good novel, or an exciting movie. ("I can't get to sleep if I'm happy, and I can't get to sleep if I'm sad; I also can't get to sleep if I'm in between and can't decide which I am.")

Phosphorus, then, is like an antenna—finely tuned to the emotional wavelength of whatever is happening around him, and open to the reception of psychic and telepathic impressions. This is the individual who sees auras or experiences déjà vu when he meets a stranger or visits an unfamiliar place. He senses the illness or death of a friend before being told of it or correctly intuits that a friend has just received some good news and telephones to ask what it is. He may also surmise the contents of a letter before opening it. One person experiences prophetic dreams; another will recount in wonder-

ful detail his encounters with the spirit world. In a house reputed to
be inhabited by a ghost, it is invariably a *Phosphorus* who will elaborate on the elusive resident's appearance and behavior.

One *Phosphorus* was staying with friends who lived in an old
rectory that, legend had it, had once been occupied by a young pastor who had lost his wife and child during an Indian raid. This was
too good an opportunity for him to miss! The next morning, at the
breakfast table, he described to his hosts and the other guests
the appearance of the ghosts of mother and child in vivid detail. The
guests exchanged knowing glances, assuming that this was his powerful imagination at work, inciting him to go one better than merely
hearing the creaking floorboards, which many others had previously
reported—until the hostess disclosed that letters existed that had
been found in the attic, in which the pastor described his wife and
child in terms almost identical with those used by the now fully vin-
dicated guest.

Any constitutional type may experience correct intuitions and
occasional brushes with the supernatural, but *Phosphorus* loves to
consider himself exceptionally endowed with psychic sensitivity and
extrasensory perception and cultivates this side of his nature.

At times the *Phosphorus* adult retains, together with a sprightly
manner and youthful looks, the spontaneity, near-innocence, and
trusting nature that is usually found only in the young. He is the free
spirit who blithely flits through life, never quite submitting to the responsibilities that come with age—a Peter Pan who resists growing
up. Thus, despite the best intentions in the world, he might find it
difficult to carry through a task, no matter how strong his original
enthusiasm. He begins on a course, then along the way a more
pressing or intriguing matter captures his notice and distracts him;
and it remains for other people to complete the work he has left unfinished.

The type may demonstrate a similar irresponsibility regarding
money—his own and others'. He generously lends or gives away
money to an admiring friend, a needy relative, or even a compara-

tive stranger. The limit of his largesse is often set only by the size of his purse, as he does not care about money per se. If he has it, he spends it like water. If he does not have it, he borrows it. If he cannot borrow it, he does without. He may also forget to repay borrowed money and believes that others should be as carefree in this matter as he is. In fact, he may be scornful of the lender for being so petty as to remember an ancient debt.

Further, like a child, *Phosphorus* can be self-centered, aware only of his own passing needs and moods. "Nobody wants me to do what I want to do, and everyone wants me to do what I *don't* want to do! I want to feel free to do what I want, when I want," was one grown woman's only half-jesting lament. Yet, here again, as with a lovable child, those around him not only indulge him, but seem almost to conspire to keep him immature. His responsive nature, winning ways, and overt gratitude toward those whom he graciously allows to spoil him encourage such humoring.

However, characteristics that are appealing in youth may lose their charm with age. Despite his sensitivity, responsiveness, and warmth—despite his talent for establishing a pleasant rapport, *Phosphorus* can be prone to edgy personal relationships and ultimately become estranged from friends, relatives, and well-wishers. As noted earlier, initially he is expert at arousing the instinctive solicitude of others, and as long as they are willing to dance to his tune, he is grateful and obliging. But once they stop dancing, he can become quarrelsome, petulant, and capricious, and somehow relations are severed. The rupture will have no discernible cause, and no one concerned will understand why it occurred—least of all *Phosphorus* himself, who is genuinely upset, even to the point of physical illness. Nevertheless, although eager in theory to do his share in maintaining relationships, he may subtly shift the burden onto others. In return for initially putting himself out for another he can, with time, grow excessively demanding of approval, approbation, and attention. In fact, he might become insistent on having his own way and being accepted for himself, defects and all ("I am the way I am. I can't change, and others must take—and love—me as I am").

There is, however, a positive aspect to all this; generally, *Phosphorus* does not bear grudges and tries not to permit ill will to be prolonged after a disagreement; nor does he usually break with people once and for all. Being by nature affectionate and wishing to return to the other's good graces, he will respond happily to overtures of reconciliation. Or he himself will initiate them, sincerely maintaining that he bears no hard feelings and trying to prevent a past friendship from dissolving into nothing.

Phosphorus is not emotionally superficial. What he professes, he genuinely feels, and feels strongly. But he might lack the steadfastness to sustain those feelings under difficult conditions. For this reason this constitutional type has been likened to a delicate blossom that thrives in the sunshine of favorable circumstances but wilts in the darkness and coldness of adversity.

Phosphorus is seldom a bookish academic. Although his initial grasp of intellectual matters is as good as anyone's and better than that of some, his mental cast is predominantly intuitive and artistic. He loves anything that captures the imagination and dislikes that which requires tedious application. Because he is quick and absorbs concepts easily, he manages to learn without applying himself too industriously. More than that: the agile, impressionable, eclectic mind, working intuitively, often comes up with something fresh or original. Thus, the type can be an excellent teacher, communicating not only with words, but also through enthusiasm and with his whole magnetic personality—and exuding that invaluable gift in a teacher, the gift of suggestion. Even if his thinking is not illuminated by trenchant logic or clarity of intellect, some truth, some insight that he throws out becomes the seed of a new thought.

Strong intuitive powers notwithstanding, *Phosphorus* can be misled by surface appearances. He does not lack discernment in his own particular field or vocation; it is when he plunges into foreign waters that his judgment flounders. His ultraimpressionable psyche is excited by too many different stimuli, and his generous nature sees too much good in too many things. Disregarding wiser counsel, he rushes into impractical ventures without thinking them through and does not easily learn that instincts, impulses, and enthusiasms must as often be controlled as encouraged. Nor does he employ the faculty of memory to gain perspective on a given situation or use it as the intellectual ballast to the emotions that it is meant to be. Ignoring the lessons of past experience, he embraces the evanescent present or his transient feelings as the entire truth—and then pursues some obviously ill-fated course of action with abandon.

Phosphorus' lack of good judgment arises in part from an overactive imagination and in part from a desire to please. These may lead him to disregard stern realities and mistake what he imagines or wishes to be true for actual fact. Thus, one woman who wished to support a benefit performance for a favorite cause, and convinced that she knew many who felt likewise committed, reserved a number of seats for the event. But on the day of the performance she arrived with only two companions—and the balance of her reserved seats went to waste. By the same token, however, when a *Phosphorus* is endowed with a strong intellect, his vivid imagination, acting in concert with an innate artistic flair, can make him a good fiction writer. In fiction, where the blend of imagination and reality is sublimated into a higher reality, the departure from prosaic truth can be brought into the service of artistic truth.

A fine example is Jane Austen, whose physical and mental traits (from the little we know of her secluded life) and literary style fit this personality type well. Contemporaries commented on her refined physical appearance and delicate features, her lustrous eyes and sparkling manner. She was a born mimic and storyteller, from an early age entertaining her family with dramatic readings from her own writings. Moreover, she died of Addison's disease, for which *Phosphorus* is one of the principal remedies.

In her novels it is Elizabeth Bennet in *Pride and Prejudice* who is the most prominently *Phosphorus* of Austen's heroines. Her vivacity and charm and wholesome optimism reflect the type's particular buoyancy and sparkle. The author's own comment on her heroine is also typical of the nature's self-appreciation: "I must confess I think her as delightful a creature as ever appeared in print; and how I shall be able to tolerate those who do not like her . . . I do not know." Furthermore, the language and style of *Pride and Prejudice* are true to type: spirited, effervescent, the wit displaying that special phosphorus-like luminescence. The author herself remarked in self-critique, "The work is rather too light, bright and sparkling: it wants shade, it wants to be stretched here and there with a long chapter of sense." In actuality, the novel's emotional subtlety and depth (the effect of its many layers of irony) exemplify *Phosphorus'* imaginative talent raised to the highest genius.

Loss of perspective, confusion of understanding, and an overactive imagination are all revealed in *Phosphorus'* love nature, especially in a woman. Not only is she a romantic who falls in love easily—and, in her willingness to be carried away by enthusiasm, is susceptible to adolescent-like crushes—but she actually cultivates the emotional soarings and plummetings that accompany being in love. Moreover, the type is starry-eyed, crediting the loved one with what she *wants* to see in him. Although this latter trait is hardly unusual in persons in an enamored state, the emotionally susceptible *Phosphorus* nourishes more extreme illusions than most. When in love, she does not remember having previously felt the same way. As with her other enthusiasms, where she tends to hail every new stimulus, idea, or gratification as a revelation, each current romance is the "real thing," and each new love is "the *most* important relationship of my life." Here, as in other spheres of life, this constitutional type would benefit from the precept "One studies history so as not to repeat it."

For her part, the woman herself, with her openly (although not necessarily consciously) enticing manner, is highly attractive to men. And certainly, this appeal is not limited to women. *Phosphorus* men can have the same inviting manner and responsive look, which is immediately felt by the opposite sex.

Similar to the restless element from which the remedy derives, the *Phosphorus* individual appears at times volatile and unsettled, without a grip on reality. Such instability might stem from the lack of a well-defined central core to the nature—that center of gravity in the psyche which sifts, sorts, and interprets impressions. In *Phosphorus,* constantly responding to his environment, the essential "I" (the selecting, binding, unifying principle) is not solid. He is a psychic sponge soaking up, almost at random, the various impressions that bombard and invade him from the external world. To such an extent might he, chameleon-like, respond to another—taking on his enthusiasms, adopting his tastes and opinions—that he grows confused as to his own identity. A not-infrequent lament is, "I don't know who I am. . . . I don't really know what I think or feel. . . . I am so busy relating to others' personalities that I lose contact with my own." In reply to Polonius' famous advice to his son (in Shakespeare's *Hamlet*), "This above all, to thine own self be true . . ." one *Phosphorus* quipped, "True to oneself—*which* self?"

Certainly, any individual undergoing stress, trauma, or major change can be confused and appear unstable, but with *Phosphorus* the condition is more chronic. He is like a bright child whose intuitions are too quick for his mind to control and whose overflow of impressions has no adequate conceptual structure to give them meaning. As a result, he can be overwhelmed by his intuitions and emotions before he has had time to arrange them in intellectual order.

The type's attractive looks and manner, self-love, self-dramatization, and natural artistry, perfectly equip *Phosphorus* for the performing arts, especially acting. Indeed, beneath his genuine sociability and talent for relating to people there often lies the love of an admiring audience (whether of one or of thousands) for whom he is prepared to supply affection and entertainment and to give his all. And because *Phosphorus,* more than any other constitutional type, is refueled by appreciation and applause, he stays on to dominate the stage and screen.

His performer's temperament compels him to be always likable, charming, magnetic—pouring himself out to his audience, both on-stage and off. And unless well disciplined in husbanding his energy and setting up emotional boundaries, he is in danger of overextension or of spreading himself too thin—of suffering from too tenuous a sense of his own identity. Like many a fine actor who is uncertain which role to play in private life, *Phosphorus* can be left somewhat disoriented when he finds himself simultaneously playing out roles and being the detached observer of his own performance.

To be sure, not all *Phosphoruses,* who are part-actors, part-spectators observing themselves perform, need to succumb to confusion of identity. A case in point is Benjamin Disraeli, twice Prime Minister of England and long-time leader of the Conservative Party. "An enigma to his contemporaries and an enigma to us today," one historian remarked, doubtless referring to the multiple facets of his personality and to his constant acting out of roles. Disraeli started out in life as an author, writing several fashionable novels about witty, foppish rising young politicians—and later seemed almost to act out the roles of his own *Phosphorus* heroes. In his political life, he wooed the staid and stolid Queen Victoria with flamboyant gallantry and exaggerated hand-kissing, and by acknowledging with tender notes (in which he called the little round tub of a woman his "faery queene") the bouquets of wildflowers that she would send him, picked by her own hands. At the same time, even while he was enjoying this performance, he always knew where he stood in the larger political scene—as he threw himself into the role of Empire Builder for his country and his Sovereign in full seriousness. Thus, he left others bemused and unable to distinguish between political genius and mere froth and surface sparkle.

This is typical of *Phosphorus.* There can be something light and airy about him, giving the impression of insubstantiality. Yet he is more complex than is suggested by his seemingly open and transparent nature. Observing him is like peering into a deep, clear pool in which everything is quite visible, even in the depths, but the shimmering play of reflected light and water allows for no true clarity.

Finally, although these pages have stressed the lively, extroverted, light-emitting personality, *Phosphorus'* shadow side must also be acknowledged. This individual, so capable of rapture and elation, so life-loving and full of sparkle, can also be prone to dark depressions. Perhaps his very ebullience and need for perpetual stimulus, excitement, or companionship are a defense against some grimly hovering specter of dejection. Certainly, his search for drama or new gratifications is a rebellion against a boredom that too easily descends on him. When the ordinary rhythms of life take their inevitable mundane course and there is insufficient color or variety in his life, *Phosphorus* succumbs to melancholy.

Altogether, *Phosphorus* is recognized in the person who displays the warm and extroverted manner of one who wants to be liked and knows how to make himself liked—who has developed a wonderful emotional receptivity and seeks to share his positive approach to existence. True, on occasion instability overrules his judgment, and he can be governed by whim, caprice, or lack of restraint. But once his emotions are stabilized and he has found a solid base or direction to his life, then this affectionate, responsive individual, with his talent for brightening others' lives, is able to reach out to many—not just to a chosen few. Such is *Phosphorus'* special gift.

Phosphorus

PRINCIPAL REGIONS AFFECTED

Head	Burning or neurologic pains, often left-sided
Throat	Dry burning pain, worse talking, coughing; laryngitis; hoarseness from overuse of voice; colds begin in the throat
Chest	Hard, dry, tight, racking, exhausting cough (that starts from a tickle in the throat and then loosens); tightness of chest or feeling as of great weight; stitches or burning in chest; expectoration has a sweetish taste; quick, oppressed breathing; pneumonia
Digestion	Sharp, cutting pains in stomach or abdomen; vomiting of food or liquid as soon as it gets warm in the stomach; liver complaints; sensation of anus remaining open after stool
Male	Sexual desire increased; complaints from sexual excesses
Female	Stress incontinence; uterine polyps; fibroids; amative disposition; weepy before menses; menses heavy, protracted; spotting between periods
Nerves	Nervous disposition; sensitive to light, sound or an inimical emotional environment; difficulty falling asleep at night because of excited state (whether happy or unhappy) or from being overstimulated by a book, movie, or interesting conversation; frequent waking; many and vivid dreams of fire, lightning, etc.; somnambulism

GENERALITIES

Tendency to bruise and bleed easily; excessive bleeding: in nosebleeds or from cuts; of gums; after tooth extraction; in tonsillectomy and other operations

Bleeding hemorrhoids, ulcers, fibroids and polyps, or blood in urine

Affections of the bones and joints

Variable internal temperature, always reacting to the climate; flushes of heat alternating with chilliness

Variable energy: high for pleasurable occupations, little energy for unpleasant ones

Sudden physical weakness when low-spirited

MODALITIES (< worse; > better)

Time	< Twilight; also morning and evening
Temperature	< Sudden changes in temperature; wind; thunderstorms
	> Cool and open air; cold bathing of face or affected parts
Position	< Lying on left or painful side
	> Lying on right side; sitting up
Food/Drink	< Salt; spicy foods
	> Cold food (salads, sandwiches) and liquids (water or carbonated drink)
	Craves salt, chocolate, ice cream, cold drinks; foods with a zesty flavor
Other	> Being rubbed, massaged, healing touch

GUIDING MENTAL SYMPTOMS

Friendly, affectionate, outgoing nature, craves companionship and approval

Fun-loving and well-disposed; but intolerant of opposition or restraint

Cheerfulness and high spirits; but under adversity can easily turn to despondency

Easily stimulated to excitement and enthusiasm

Highly impressionable; sensitive to what is seen, heard, or read

Fanciful imagination

Telepathic abilities

Artistic mentality; remedy picture frequently encountered among actors and other performing artists

Fears abandonment and being alone; the dark, robbers; misfortune, impending disease, death; thunder and lightning; also free-floating anxieties

Calcarea carbonica

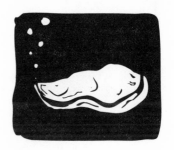

C alcarea carbonica is the potentized carbonate of lime, taken from the middle layer of the oyster shell. The images evoked by this mollusk are the following: first, the animal itself—cold, pale, moist, limp, inactive; second, the shell—thick, impenetrable, fixed to a rock, protecting the completely defenseless creature within; third, within this otherwise undistinguished creature there grows a pearl of polished and delicate beauty, born through steady concretion around an irritating grain of sand. Keeping in mind these three images, the oyster itself, the shell, and the pearl, we will examine how they relate to the *Calcarea* individual.

The inactive oyster, firmly attached to its rock, is the most passive member of the mollusk family. Correspondingly, the *Calcarea* personality type, on the physical level, tends to display a slow metabolism, a sluggish circulation, flabby muscle tone (often with limp, moist extremities), and an overall lack of endurance. He is chilly, worse from exertion, and even mild physical effort leaves him perspiring and out of breath. The same placid nature is reflected on the mental level in the individual who is lethargic, often phlegmatic, neither easily aroused nor easily moved, and content to do the barest minimum. From disinclination for work or because mental exertion fatigues him, it may take him a day or more to accomplish what oth-

ers do in a couple of hours. Or he begins a course of study, but then
cannot complete it; somewhere along the way he feels resistant to
being intellectually pressured or otherwise stressed or overworked.
The words "stressed" or "overworked," however, are relative. What
is stressful to *Calcarea* might be a part of another's normal routine.
To this inactive individual any additional exertion can be felt as too
much effort and, even if pleasurable, raises the question, "Is it worth
the bother?" Moreover, it is hard for him to imagine others even
wanting to do that which is an effort to him.

Calcarea's inertia is rooted not only in a dislike of being forced
to exert himself but also in an absence of ambition, energy, and
drive. He considers striving and hard work to be as unnecessary to
himself as they are distasteful. Therefore, leaving aside spiritual or
moral worth and judging by purely worldly standards, he may be
seen as unsuccessful because he will not push or compete in a
world in which a certain amount of pushing and competition is required. This personality type might even retain the immaturity or
undeveloped quality of a child—and often wants to remain a child,
preferring its slow, protected, tranquil existence to the striving, competitive world of adulthood. In fact, in its unequaled role as pro-
moter of healthy physical and mental growth in the young child,
Calcarea carbonica is homoeopathy's sovereign children's remedy.
Thus, the theme of "the child" crops up periodically in an analysis of
this archetype.

In *Calcarea* one encounters the classic procrastinator. "Why do
today what can be put off until tomorrow?" is his subliminal philosophy, and he allows himself to be distracted from paying bills, writing the important letter, making the necessary telephone calls. Or, he
tarries and fiddles with little things, wearing himself out with minutiae, so as to postpone undertaking the larger task. The individual
aspiring to be a writer starts his day by wandering around the house,
picking up dishes and rinsing out ashtrays, sorting out old papers or
pottering around in the garden, until he has so depleted his energy
that the whole day is wasted as far as serious writing is concerned.

Students are chronically unprepared in class or unable to submit papers on time, asking for extensions. The housewife procrastinates with her chores, the husband with his house repairs until, overwhelmed by the accumulated responsibilities, *Calcarea* finds himself in the unwelcome situation of having to operate under pressure and then worrying about all the things he should be doing in life, but is not.

Under stress, *Calcarea*'s mind easily becomes confused. Difficulty in collecting his thoughts and in finding the right words and expressions are among the most common manifestations (for instance, he will say, "I am leaving for New York"—where he is at present—when he means "Boston"). One person cannot recollect what was just spoken or what he has just read, or comes up with a different number every time he adds up a column of figures; another person cannot recall what he has to do today or enters a room and forgets why he has come; while yet another cannot recall where he has put things. Confusion and poor concentration are occasionally reflected in his rambling conversation, where he either branches off into areas only marginally related to the question asked or takes a long time getting to the point. Yet, just as a child who is seemingly in his own world, not following the drift of conversation, suddenly makes a perceptive remark, so the adult, with his somewhat crablike mind, eventually works round to the point and contributes a comment of rare insight.

Even in the individual who seems ambitious and determined to succeed, the *Calcarea carbonica* pattern may be discerned. As the oyster imperceptibly adds layer upon layer to form a pearl, so this person works slowly and conscientiously, piling stone upon stone. Thus, a writer might spend his entire life on one novel or a single collection of essays, while the efforts of your true *Calcarea* plodder may never come to light at all. Emblematic of this latter type is the kindly old headmaster, Dr. Strong, in Dickens' *David Copperfield,* with his childlike simplicity, guilelessness, and interminable "Dictionary of Greek Roots," which, *Calcarea*-like, never gets written beyond the letter *D.* Characteristic also is his limp handshake, which

Dickens ingeniously describes: ". . . and then he gave me his hand which I didn't know what to do with as it did nothing for itself."

There exists, however, an interesting and often-encountered variant of *Calcarea*'s inability to complete a work, and that is the inability to *begin* it. To muster up the energy to get going takes a major effort, but once he begins—once his imagination has been stimulated by the job—then, like an enthralled child, he cannot tear himself away. He may even become the immoderate worker, who perseveres with unswerving pertinacity, to compensate for a fundamental lethargy. This diligence can sometimes reach the point where he works all day without letup, barely stopping for meals, for fear that once he does stop he will not be able to regain momentum. In a word, *Calcarea,* in his work habits, finds it difficult to pace himself—fluctuating between indolence and exaggerated industry.

The *Calcarea carbonica* nature is a vulnerable one (think of the vulnerability of the oyster's soft body). He is slow to rebound from emotional shock, is sensitive to criticism, and lacks confidence in his own capacities. The student in school is so fearful of failing that he is unable to study, and his worst apprehensions are confirmed. The woman feels incompetent or slower compared with others, and is so flurried when she has to perform that the incompetence she fears becomes a reality. A man worries about acquitting himself honorably at his job. A columnist with fifteen years' experience and an excellent body of work might still be fearful of criticism every time his editor calls him in to his office to consult with him. Generally speaking, this insecure individual is apprehensive of being wounded by quicker, sharper minds or of being imposed on by stronger personalities. The type is encountered in the offspring of famous or forceful parents who tend to overshadow their children and (even if unwittingly) prevent them from fully developing their own characters or finding their own paths. The son who automatically succeeds to his father's business or profession, whether or not he has any inclination or natural aptitude for it, is frequently a *Calcarea carbonica*.

Other fears of this constitutional type are of the dark; of bugs and crawly things in general, or some particular rodent, reptile, or insect; of ill-health, especially ailments of the heart; or of impending misfortune. This last anxiety even expresses itself vicariously in a profound dislike of hearsay or newspaper accounts of grief or violence. It is especially true of the *Calcarea* woman; if she hears or reads something upsetting, she is unable to get the unpleasantness out of her mind. Therefore, she will not listen to the news on radio or television and refuses to read the daily paper. Even a man of the world might refuse to look at war movies or read a book depicting cruelty; the impression is too debilitating and too lasting. In general, because *Calcarea* feels deeply (the oyster resides in the very depths of the ocean) impressions stay with him a long time.

But, above all, *Calcarea* dreads new challenges and enterprising new starts. He dislikes change, fears upheavals, and prefers even a monotonous existence to venturing forth into the unknown. His present life may be restricted, even difficult, but at least it is less psychologically intimidating than an unfamiliar new one. An example of the type's oysterlike clinging to the parent rock was the elderly gentleman who had been a bank teller his whole life. He had remained at the same bank, almost at the same window, for nearly half a century, never receiving a promotion or even a raise in salary beyond automatic increases. He had, earlier in his career, been offered a more responsible post but had turned it down, being perfectly content with his old position, at which he stayed well beyond the usual age for retirement.

In addition to lack of enterprise, *Calcarea* might exhibit a fear of succeeding. When things are going well, the student in graduate school, the woman rising in her profession, the man thriving in business is suddenly overwhelmed by the responsibility and throws it all over—and either drifts away or goes back to a less challenging occupation.

We now turn to the hard, protective shell in which the oyster's soft, defenseless body is encased. The principal defense of a vulnerable creature against an inimical or intrusive environment or against the stronger beings that surround him is to withdraw into himself; and this, indeed, is one of *Calcarea*'s principal defensive reactions. To protect his sensitive psyche he retires into his shell, closing off and ignoring the world. He is not necessarily shy or timid—intrinsically he is of a sociable disposition, and he also possesses a quiet, philosophical assurance—but he sees how the outside world operates and decides that it is not for him.

Predictably, then, this is the person who will be strongly attached to the home (to the most familiar) and clings to everything related to it. In families with a heavy *Calcarea carbonica* component, the members like nothing better than to gather around and enjoy each other's company, appreciating the closeness of being at home together. They do not seek adventures or go out and *do* things, but are content with that which seems from the outside a uniform, uneventful life; yet to them it is a rich and rewarding one. *Calcarea* may actually feel nervous and uneasy when away from the physical proximity of home or the street on which he lives. One man joked about his wife, "Whenever we are away from home and driving back, she's in such a hurry that I can hardly persuade her to let me stop for gas!" This kind of disorientation is reminiscent of the oyster, which cannot survive without its protective shell.

As a result, *Calcarea*'s outlook may be restricted. A *Calcarea* woman, for example, may be incapable of raising her sights above complicated and all too frequently trifling family relationships: who quarreled with whom or what one member said to another. She does not offer solutions or consider any effective course of action for settling the discord, but harps on what she has seen or heard in a helpless, hopeless way. At times, flustered and unaware of any other method of resolving her troubles than by talking of them, she repeats the same sentiment, the same phrases, such as, "Oh, I wish such and such had [or had not] happened!"—pointlessly, since it has not [or has already] taken place. She does not let go even at night and lies awake churning over in her mind some worrying thought. The fretting *Calcarea*, in fact, invites the admonition, "Put it aside!

The world is larger than your own back yard." But her instinctive response to such a charge would be, "What *is* more important than the small things in family relations that make life either pleasant or disagreeable?" Significantly, however, *Calcarea* does not magnify the importance of a particular event for effect; there is no desire to astound. She merely magnifies its importance to herself.

A characteristic related to the restricted outlook is this constitutional type's easy philosophical resignation to whatever he decides he cannot alter about his life. Serene acceptance of one's fate is a precious possession, but when carried too far, this quality, reinforced by an inherent lack of enterprise, can develop into defeatism. "What is fated to be will be. What is the use of opposing destiny?" *Calcarea* reasons, refusing to make any effort to change or improve a situation.

A fine literary portrayal of the type's fatalism, restrictive outlook, and withdrawing into his shell is found in the Russian novel *Oblomov* by Ivan Goncharov. The hero, Ilya Oblomov, is a lethargic but sensitive, unexciting but pleasant-mannered, gentleman, who takes 200 pages (one third of the novel) just to get out of bed in the morning and put on his bathrobe. This slow-paced opening scene symbolizes the nature of the man and of his subsequent life. Resisting all the energizing efforts of his active friend, Stoltz, Oblomov prefers to sleep and dream rather than get up and take an interest in the world. Also, as the flashbacks in the novel reveal, he is attempting to recreate his happy childhood and the leisurely, peaceful, carefree contentment he knew growing up at his mother's knee. Through apathy, procrastination, and refusal to rise to an emotional challenge Oblomov loses the woman he loves (and who loves him) to the energetic Stoltz. But he accepts the loss with typical *Calcarea* resignation, sinking back into his habitual indolence. For the rest of his life he remains ensconced in his pleasantly stagnant morass of a home, as placidly content with his limited existence as an oyster on a rock.

In shielding himself from the world's pressures, *Calcarea* may refuse to respond to the exigencies of time. Engrossed in something of interest, he can lose track of time altogether. "I'll *just* finish read-

ing this article," he thinks, "and then I'll run that errand." Then he
"just" forgets. He wants to stop by the post office on the way to an
appointment, but starts chatting with a friend there, and the time
passes faster than he realizes. Unconcerned with punctuality, he can
be habitually late to the theater, to weddings, religious services,
classes, concerts, and so on. One man who loved music and theater
stated that in a long marriage he and his *Calcarea* wife arrived on
time to a cultural event only once—the opera *Rigoletto*; and for a
time her lateness was almost grounds for divorce. "However," he
added, "I've come to realize that being late is not the end of the
world. But [with a wistful sigh] I do hope that *some* day before I die
I'll be able to see the first act of *Hamlet,* hear the first movement of
my favorite piano concertos, and learn exactly *what* happens in the
first half of the ballet *Giselle*. I've seen her come to life in the underworld three times and still don't know why she died."

Just as *Calcarea* is the last to arrive, so he may be the last to
leave. Once settled at a gathering, he sees no reason to depart and
stays on and on. There is a saying that some individuals leave without saying "goodbye," whereas others say "goodbye" and do not
leave. *Calcarea* belongs definitely to the latter class. Quite oblivious
of the time and in his enjoyment in talking, he will stand in the door-
way for an hour bidding his host goodnight.

Perhaps the most prominent of *Calcarea*'s shell-like protective
techniques against too much external pressure is obstinacy—a trait
encountered even in the basically well-behaved child and good-
natured adult. Seemingly compliant and easy-going, he might be impossible to move; he simply digs in his heels and refuses to budge.
As one woman said of her obliging, roly-poly husband, "Sure, he
looks like a cream puff, but *no one* pushes him around!" Or, an employer will tell his *Calcarea* secretary to type letters in a particular
way. Doggedly, and without arguing, she will continue typing them
the same way as before. He can rant and rave, but to little avail; he
is quite helpless confronted with her stubborn resistance. Admit-
tedly, there is something in the intractable, balky individual that invites criticism and incites others to push or try to change him. But in

his impassive, unyielding way he resists even the strongest pressure, holding steadfastly to his position. Attempts to make him respond are like trying, without a special knife, to pry open the shell of a reluctant oyster. This nonaggressive yet determined obstinacy gives the impression of slowness or denseness; actually, it is a weaker-positioned individual's most effective defense against more powerful forces or personalities surrounding him.

The highest potential of the oyster is to form a perfect, lustrous pearl; but if the critical grain of sand is not introduced into its amorphous organism, the pearl remains unformed. By the same token, if *Calcarea* as a child is deprived of a necessary irritating stimulus, he may, as an adult, remain undeveloped or unfulfilled.

Some types—shrewd, wily street-urchins—can mature on their own. Throw them out into the world, and they flourish. They are self-motivated, savvy, resourceful, and extract lessons from whatever experience life offers—hardy wildflowers that survive by the roadside or weeds that spring up through the cracks in city sidewalks.

Calcarea carbonica, however, is a hothouse plant that needs careful and systematic cultivation to thrive. He cannot develop by himself but demands structured, and preferably individualized, guidance. This characteristic, in an extreme form, is exemplified in the education of Wolfgang Amadeus Mozart and Helen Keller. Both were gifted and receptive *Calcarea* types, who responded to the steady irritation of an outside influence—their resolute teachers, Leopold Mozart and Annie Sullivan. The stories are legendary of how these two driving forces devoted their own considerable gifts and energies almost exclusively to cultivating the talents of their young charges—relentlessly steering them to greatness.

Little is known of Mozart's life, especially his childhood, but that he early showed signs of being a *Calcarea carbonica* is attested to in his infant intolerance of milk—even that of his mother and a wet nurse—which necessitated a diet of gruel from birth and made his very survival a miracle. While indubitably of independent disposition, he was yet, up until the age of eighteen, remarkably amenable to parental authority, allowing his every step to be guided by his ambitious father. Thereafter, whatever traits of other constitutional remedies Mozart displayed as an adult, he definitely retained a *Calcarea* immaturity in the sense of being financially naive, thoughtless of the future, and childish in behavior to the point of eccentricity.

Helen Keller's life, by contrast, is well documented. She was a typically *Calcarea carbonica* child: of stocky build, with wavy blond hair and full red cheeks, who from an early age was prone to high fevers, one of which deprived her of sight and hearing when she was only eighteen months old. During the five years that elapsed between her illness and the appearance of her teacher on the scene, she manifested no particular intelligence or curiosity (her sole interest being food) and made little progress in understanding the dark, silent world she inhabited. Not only did she give no indication of the genius she was later to display, but was even considered mentally retarded. Her stubbornness was notorious. Before the arrival of Annie Sullivan, no one could influence her; her teacher's hardest task was to break through the child's resistance to being taught. True to type, she was at first slow to catch on. Although nearly seven, she took many weeks to understand that there was a relationship between the outside world and the impressions her teacher was making on her hand. Once launched, however, her steady, lifelong accrual of knowledge and remarkable accomplishments under the systematic guidance of Annie Sullivan (learning several languages, graduating with honors from Radcliffe College, writing about important social and world issues, and lecturing around the world) never halted.

Without a strong and steady outside guidance, however, *Calcarea* may not be motivated to stretch his mind or seek new forms and experiences, as the development of talent requires. Often he is satisfied to remain a man of activities in lieu of becoming a man of action—a dabbler who refuses to enter on a serious venture because of the rigor of its demands. He remains the spontaneous and unselfconsciously creative child, who takes up one interest after another, enjoying each, but never committing himself entirely to any one.

The young adult, for example, might be forever switching areas of study, never finding one suited to his particular needs. Thus, this constitutional type is discerned in the original, *sui generis* mind that has never been properly disciplined or directed—in the gifted, amateur mentality. However (and since this is a prominent feature, it is worth reiterating), where another would feel oppressed because not fulfilling his potential, *Calcarea* is resigned—and perfectly content.

Certainly, on occasion, one does encounter the reverse side of this lack of drive. Sensing the need for more formal guidance ("After having been a drifter for thirty-five years, I suddenly realized that I know nothing from nothing"), the mature *Calcarea* might at some point begin deliberately to impose structure on himself by going back to college, which he had dropped out of many years ago, or in other ways subjecting himself to a strict systematic discipline and hard work. Then it is that an unexpectedly beautiful pearl is brought forth. This craving for rigorous discipline is encountered even in the young. An example is the *Calcarea* high school student who stayed up nights writing sonnets, sestinas, rondelets, and mock epics in heroic couplets for her English composition course. When asked if she had been assigned these difficult poetic forms, she replied that the class was allowed to write in any form they chose—and that she used to write in blank verse, but that it was too easy. She now chose these highly structured forms to make it harder; also because, "By trying to find rhymes and forcing myself to adhere to a certain rhythm, I find myself looking for new ideas and new words, and this makes me discover thoughts that I *never knew I had!*"

In this connection it is worth noting that because of the low-key quality of his virtues or abilities—because he is generally free from boastfulness, presumption, or desire for display—*Calcarea* himself is often unaware of the pearl he is harboring. With feelings deeper than he can or is willing to express, in social situations he tends to play the role not of a star, but of the passive, nonjudgmental observer. Perhaps his distinguishing feature is allowing others to be themselves—just as *he* wishes to be allowed to be himself. This fellow-sympathy, coupled with an ability to sense others' feelings and thoughts at their most profound, renders him appreciative of qualities in a person that others may not perceive or understand.

Calcarea's respect for others' personalities and idiosyncrasies, together with his quickness in sensing their hidden virtues, goes hand-in-hand with a desire to nurture; for this type is by nature a nurturer. Even on the material level it is he, or especially she, who insists on plying others with food and drink on every possible occasion and who displays an exceptional talent for hospitality. Everything flows smoothly and naturally at her gatherings, where food is plentiful and others feel at ease in the warm, comfortable, friendly atmosphere of a nonpressured environment. The *Calcarea* individual is happy to oblige in this or in any other way he can. Others gravitating to him for nurture are welcome to what he has to give. Nor does he expect reciprocity. There is a self-sufficiency (or privacy) about him that asks little of others in return and prefers to keep his own counsel. Just as an individual of solitary tendencies might choose to live anonymously in a crowded city, so *Calcarea* surrounds himself with people in an attempt to remain relatively inconspicuous in a group and preserve his privacy.

Calcarea carbonica is recognized in the somewhat placid, at times plodding, often insecure individual whose virtues and talents, even if considerable, remain low-key—unless he is prodded to high achievement by some outside force. The type is also recognized in one whose whole being cries out for guidance, structure, and discipline so that he may become less lethargic, less unformed, or more fulfilled in his potential. And because of the remedy's capacity to address these traits as well as many of the unresolved fears and insecurities of childhood, the undistinguished gray shell of the lowly oyster can rightly be regarded as one of nature's greatest homoeopathic gifts to humanity.

Calcarea carbonica

PRINCIPAL REGIONS AFFECTED

Head　　Easy fatigue of the eyes; chronically stuffed nose; face pallid, pasty, and puffy

Chest　　Palpitations (especially at night); shortness of breath; **coughs**, with burning and soreness in the chest; troublesome at night and with expectoration only during the day

Digestion　**Impaired nutrition is the keynote to many complaints,** contributing to **faulty bone and teeth development; constipation (but without discomfort),** also diarrhea of undigested food, stomach pains, and other forms of poor digestion

Female　　Fibroids; **menses too early, too long, too profuse, brought on early by excitement or getting chilled; sore, swollen breasts before menses;** problems during lactation; milk either too profuse, scanty or absent; distasteful to child; difficulties weaning

Nerves　　Restless sleep with frequent waking; **disagreeable ideas running through the head prevent sleep or rouse from light sleep;** nightmares: dreams of monsters, snakes, etc.

GENERALITIES

Looks well-fed and robust, but is not strong

Weak, flabby muscle tone; poor physical and mental stamina; low energy

Perspires easily on exertion, especially on head or chest; during sleep

Sour odor to perspiration, eructations, diarrhea; sour taste in mouth

Unhealthy looking skin

Cannot tolerate pressure of clothes, especially around waist and abdomen

Continued.

Calcarea carbonica—cont'd

MODALITIES (< worse; > better)

Time	< Awakening; full moon
Temperature	< Cold: raw, damp air, cold bathing, cooling off after being heated; change of weather to cold
	> Warmth: of sun, room, clothes; warm dry climate
Energy	< Mental or physical exertion (especially when ascending stairs, hills, etc.)
	> Sedentary pursuits
Food/Drink	< Milk, eggs
	Craves sweets, dairy, creamy foods, carbohydrates, eggs; may have an aversion to meat
	> Simple bland food
Other	< Hearing or reading of cruelty or violence

GUIDING MENTAL SYMPTOMS

Outwardly placid and phlegmatic, but inwardly sensitive and vulnerable

Mind easily confused

Tired or jaded mental state with disinclination for work

Indolence; procrastination; but once engrossed, might have difficulty letting up

Conscientious and reliable once committed

Independent-minded

Inordinate obstinacy, even while good natured

Many anxieties and apprehensions: fears insects, mice, or reptiles; the dark; contagious disease or heart ailments; death; loss of mental powers; poverty; misfortune; the safety and security of loved ones and the home; leaving home, new beginnings; success; being overwhelmed

Lycopodium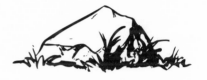

L ycopodium is the clubmoss, whose spores are shaped like a wolf's paw; hence the origin of the Greek name: *lyco* (wolf) and *podos* (foot). Moss is one of the oldest plant life forms on earth, having existed since the Devonian period some 370 million years ago; yet it has survived essentially unchanged despite all the intervening geological cataclysms and climatic upheavals. Its lovely green is restful to the eye and soothing to the spirit; its resilient softness is cooling to the touch; and its pertinacious growth throughout the ages suggests an indestructible nature. The associations thus evoked by the moss family are serenity and stability.

As we seek correspondences between the plant and the man, we find that *Lycopodium* possesses a pleasant and self-contained personality, soothing in its composure and self-possession and, at least outwardly, stable and balanced. He is temperate by inclination and in his measured lifestyle, seldom overextends himself emotionally; and in his capacity to adapt to changing scenes and varying environments without himself mutating in the process, one senses an undercurrent of quiet strength.

One of the more striking characteristics of the *Lycopodium* male (and it is the male who is primarily addressed in this chapter) is his self-esteem. He has the air of one who obviously has a good opinion of himself, is confident in his own judgment, and believes that he knows best at all times. He considers himself an example of reasonableness and moderation others would do well to follow and is convinced that the world would be a far, far better place if it contained more right-thinking and right-acting persons like himself. Such high self-esteem is bound to win the esteem of others. Indeed, his very character, behavior, and assurance all inspire respect. Moreover, he is psychologically astute in making himself liked as well as respected by means of a gracious and courteous manner that almost imperceptibly brings others under his will.

Lycopodium's self-esteem is strengthened by his conviction that he was born under a lucky star. Life seems to encourage him in this feeling. Focused and self-disciplined, he succeeds easily in his career and personal as well as professional relations. He trusts to his good fortune, hopes for the best and, with his sanguine outlook and innate competence, his ventures do tend to work out well. If not, it is no great matter; resilient and robust, he goes on to the next thing. All this enhances his seeming invulnerability and further reinforces his high opinion of himself.

In dealing with the world at large, *Lycopodium* appears full of faith in humanity, but beneath his open and pleasant manner he often harbors caution and mistrust, with little faith in anyone but himself. In his heart he is a skeptic who expects little of frail and erring mortals. He is convinced that others cannot do things nearly as well as he and always relies on himself to perform better. Yet caution and skepticism do not make him fault finding; they make him pragmatic. In dealing with people, he does not hold them to too-high standards but remains essentially realistic about their limitations and works well with whatever material is at hand.

Accepting people as they are without being unduly critical facilitates smooth and easy relationships. He is neither easily disappointed in others nor hurt by them. He is tolerant of mediocrity and even of inferiority in those around him and, outside his immediate family, he does not try to change them. Because of this, others, sensing that *Lycopodium* does not expect more than they can or are willing to give, feel comfortable with him—all of which contributes to his social resilience.

However, his skepticism and mistrust, combined with a tendency to magnify his own abilities, can lead him to one of his consistent intellectual weaknesses: underrating others' capacities and underestimating his competitors, peers, family, and even friends. The half-mocking lament, "Oh, what a trying fate it is to be always right, when others are so wrong!" reveals his true mindset. Thus is laid the groundwork for the special *Lycopodium* arrogance. It is he, of all types, who suffers most from that flaw of the heroes of Greek tragedy, *hubris*: a short-sighted intellectual pride that darkens the understanding.

Lycopodium may feel so obviously in the right that he will often refuse even to discuss a matter. In the middle of an argument, and especially if the other has made a strong point, he gets up and walks away. Like a stately ambassador, ignoring his adversary's challenges, he senses the moment to withdraw from an unproductive situation and retreat with honor. And when he does deign to engage in contention, he can be a master of evasion, clever at avoiding direct confrontation on the enemy's own territory. He subtly retreats from hostile ground by eluding the central issue, deflecting the argument, or changing the subject. Then he pulls his opponent deeper into his own terrain, where he can more easily rout him. On the rare occasions when he does admit to being mistaken in an argument, his tone conveys the cavalier attitude, "All right, all right, have it your own way, if you *do* insist," implying that because the other party is being completely unreasonable, he himself is capitulating magnanimously.

Just as *Lycopodium* tries to avoid argument, he will avoid rupturing relationships. Discord or breaking with others is undignified and beneath his self-respect. It tarnishes his image of being able to get along with anyone, of understanding everyone, and of being respected by all; and he will bend over backward not to estrange himself from family, associates, friends, and subordinates.

In the professional field, he will try to patch up disagreements with an adversary or competitor by having a friendly drink and talking things over in a tactful, conciliatory manner. No type is better at separating personal feelings from professional. He can engage in heated debate with an opponent in the courts, the boardroom, or the smoke-filled chambers of political life, and be laughing and joking with him an hour later. Calling a cease-fire, he puts aside professional rivalry and sincerely enjoys the company of his adversary. And it is the capable *Lycopodium* employer who is reluctant to dismiss incompetent employees. He would rather retain them than sever relationships and create bad feelings. Even after a bitter divorce, it is important for the type's self-esteem to remain on amicable terms with his ex-wife and in-laws.

This is an attractive trait. *Lycopodium* is ready to overlook past discord and does not harbor resentments. Possessing a healthy "That's water over the dam" attitude, he looks forward to starting anew. His conscious or unconscious philosophy is that more is achieved by mending than by breaking—by conciliation than by antagonism. Believing that to forgive is wisdom but to forget is sublime, he makes a point of maintaining social harmony by forgiving and forgetting.

Just as the resilient moss conforms to the configuration of the landscape and the changing environment, while proceeding undaunted along its way, so *Lycopodium* displays a viability that stems from a resolute yet supple nature that permits him to adapt to fluctuating times and shifting scenes while pursuing his own policies. When circumstances change and he is forced to change an opinion he does not become confused, but remains buoyant. He justifies his inconsistencies with "What I said yesterday was yesterday. Today is different."

It does not automatically follow that *Lycopodium* is exploitative or self-serving. Although he can be competitive and jealous of his position, striving for power and prestige, he also possesses a keen sense of service and sincerely wants to make a good job of his life. Taking pride in work that is well done and beneficial to humanity, he often devotes himself to it unsparingly. In fact, he may derive his greatest security and deepest satisfaction—his very identity, even— from his profession. But he is able to run with the hare one day and hunt with the hounds the next, because his strongest loyalty is to his own viability.

This last trait is strengthened by his particular understanding of "truth." He is the individual who would ask with Pontius Pilate, "What is Truth?" suggesting that the question has no answer—and that today's truth is but tomorrow's error. In other words, he embraces the diplomat's or politician's conviction that truth is variable and flexible. There can be truth only for a given situation, for a given person, at a given moment. Proceeding from this premise, he then coolly adapts his idea of truth to the temper of the times.

Therefore, *Lycopodium* does not always tell the objective truth. He prefers to tell people what they want to hear, what they are prepared to hear, or, above all, what he thinks they should hear. To ask whether he is truthful is to ask the wrong question: he is, and he is not. He is frankly convinced that the end justifies the means and that every person must engage in some untruths for the sake of an ultimate goal. When challenged, he will openly admit to an elastic mentality, explaining that times and circumstances alter and that he is consequently forced to modify his opinions. Anyone in a position of power or authority acts on this principle to some extent and learns to respect it, but with *Lycopodium* the conviction is instinctive and is reflected in all his motives, actions, and relationships—personal as well as professional.

The French diplomat and statesman Talleyrand comes to mind as the quintessential viable *Lycopodium*. A bishop under the Bourbon monarchy, an ambassador under the Girondins, Grand Chamberlain under Napoleon, and Foreign Minister under the restored Bourbon regime, Talleyrand was hardly a paragon of consistency. It required no common mental elasticity, not to mention diplomatic ability and tact, to hold leading positions under four different forms of French government without forfeiting his credibility. It was at the Congress of Vienna, however, after the Napoleonic Wars, that Talleyrand best exhibited his incomparable *Lycopodium* gifts of shrewd statesmanship. Despite much opposition to his very presence there, the French envoy insinuated his way into the graces of the participating dignitaries, as they fought each other for power and precedence, convincing them all that an intact and prosperous France was to their political advantage. Thus he steered his country through the Congress without loss of territory or prestige. Later in life, when criticized for the apparent elasticity of his loyalties and principles, Talleyrand would state that he never abandoned any government before it abandoned itself, but he did so just a little earlier than other people, as his watch was a little fast.

Simultaneously (and paradoxically) *Lycopodium* can display a deep, strong conservative bent of mind. He may be reluctant to change his job or residence, even if it means leaving a worse situation for a better one. He prefers to live where he has always lived; despite changes of fashion, wear clothes he has always worn; and continue to do what he has always done. This quality, arising primarily from caution and circumspection, makes up part of his complexity. He is undeniably adaptable on the intellectual or abstract planes; his psyche easily adjusts to changing ideas and circumstances in the world at large; but he is also unyieldingly set in his ways and tenaciously conservative in all that concerns him personally (his habits, diet, health, family, and so on). Furthermore, although in major upheavals *Lycopodium* exhibits remarkable equanimity, calmly accepting severe reversals (in a crisis he is magnificent: cool, supportive, reliable), small changes can throw him completely off-balance. For instance, he is one of the few personality types to be actively upset by the disposal of an old dishrag, worn out and full of holes. Others may hang on to the rag out of economy, but *Lycopodium*'s motive is different (although he, too, hates being wasteful). It is his innate conservatism (i.e., tenacity) that is disturbed by losing something to which he has grown accustomed. "I liked the old dishrag," he may say in annoyance. "I knew where the holes were and worked around them. I don't *want* a change of

kitchen rag at this stage of my life. Why [turning on the culprit in ir-
ritation] did you throw it away? And why is everyone *always* working against me the moment my back is turned?"

Lycopodium's mosslike indestructibility permits him to operate
well even in a hostile environment; experiences or events that devastate others (such as a difficult childhood) do not devastate him.
However, one organism's viability is often exercised or attained at
the expense of another. Even if unobtrusively, the more viable will
trespass on the terrain of the less viable, causing the latter to suffer.

In just such a way, *Lycopodium* oppresses weaker persons close
to him, particularly his spouse and children. Avoiding the stronger
organisms he cannot dominate, he often chooses a gentle, self-effac-
ing, or sickly spouse—who is satisfied to be guided entirely by her
husband and prepared to play the role of "the wife" in their married
life. He is able to elicit the most extraordinary devotion; his wife
lives almost solely for his needs, and both partners are content. A
woman who was asked how her marriage had survived so long, and
who replied, "It is because we have both been in love with the same
man for thirty-five years," surely had a *Lycopodium* for a husband.
Trouble begins only when the wife, tired of playing second fiddle,
wants recognition in her own right.

The type's oppression of those around him has yet another
facet. Quite unconsciously he may encourage—even create—inferiority in others. His very competence and outward strength elicit the
opposite qualities in those who are close. It is not easy to live in
the shadow of someone who is always self-assured, always in command, always gracious in public—and always right. Others may be
excused for giving up the struggle when confronted with so much
viability. Since much of this dialectic is acted out on the subconscious levels (the sense of superiority is innate to the type) it is not
only concealed from the average outsider but for the longest time
usually goes unrecognized by the principals involved. *Lycopodium*
himself is certainly unaware of his influence, and the immediate
family only vaguely senses that something is draining them of initia-

tive. This overbearing individual can operate so imperceptibly, so like a soft blanket of moss, that the family members little suspect what is smothering them.

In many spheres, in fact, *Lycopodium* courts inferiors and surrounds himself with them. Of the competent he is, at times, overly critical, even suspicious; while inferiors bring out all his magnanimity. He loves to feel generous, understanding, forgiving, and tolerant toward erring or weaker mortals. After all, the dullness or incompetence of others permits him to shine the brighter. Also, of course, inferiors are nonthreatening. They will not challenge his insecurities and are unlikely to surprise him in some weakness or misstep. Consciously or unconsciously *Lycopodium* is always protecting his image of strength and invincibility.

Another prominent *Lycopodium* characteristic is detachment, a feeling he cultivates at almost any cost. Aloof from the turmoils of earth, he likes to float somewhere above struggling humanity, unruffled and unperturbed, regarding it from the lofty perspective of his detachment. He is interested, ready to advise and to help, but refuses to be emotionally involved—realizing that his viability depends to some degree on emotional distance. To such an extent does he place a dignified distance between himself and unwelcome worldly concerns that when something disagreeable, undesirable, or unacceptable does arise, he may not confront it. Others encountering a problem say to themselves, "Here is a problem; now, how do I deal with it?" *Lycopodium,* rejecting whatever might disturb his detachment, says, "Here is a problem; now, how do I *avoid* it?"

A classic technique that may be used to remain detached is humor. Wit is a notorious substitute for emotion, and resorting to humor is a time-honored way of preserving emotional aloofness. Speaking of *Lycopodium,* a friend or relation will say, "He keeps me at a distance with his joking manner"; or "He always makes a joke of an important matter, which dismisses it." Certainly, *Lycopodium* does enjoy relating to people on a surface, joking basis—and often excels in light conversation and sophisticated small talk at large gatherings where strangers mix and exchange witticisms, while the emotional demands remain negligible.

His humor can be described as "wry," reflecting an innate urbanity and dispassionate mentality. At times he assumes that irritating tone of one who is detached from himself, knows and sees through himself, but does not expect others to do so. He is willing enough to make self-deprecatory remarks but will not permit others to laugh at his expense. Highly conscious of power, and well aware that wit is power, he prefers to wield that weapon himself. At another's joke he will smile reluctantly, with the characteristic *Lycopodium* guarded or half-smile, or will produce a repartee or counterjoke of his own and only then laugh.

A pleasant bearing and good manners can be another form of substitute for strong feelings. If a person assumes a proper look of concern, he need not become emotionally involved. In this sphere *Lycopodium* possesses consummate skill. Both socially and professionally, he can listen attentively and intelligently to the problems of others without taking things too much to heart. His very reserve is reassuring. Behind the self-contained and understated manner lies a hint—a promise, even, that he could give more if he chose.* But, that he remains ultimately untouched, that his sincere interest lasts only as long as the other person is present, becomes apparent when, a few days later, he has completely forgotten what the other said. When the same conversation with the same person is repeated all over again, it is news to him. Although his memory might be jogged and he might think to himself, "Hmm—how interesting! It somehow

---

*Like the man, the *Lycopodium* woman may exhibit an incomparable skill in dealing with people in both her personal and professional life. Unfazed by demanding family, clients, or colleagues, she remains collected, pleasant, even-tempered—suave and self-possessed at all times and under all circumstances. The woman who is able to keep her distance while demonstrating the care and concern of a true friend, and who displays a gift of tact and diplomacy bordering on genius, is bound to have *Lycopodium* in her constitutional picture.

rings a bell. Now, *where* did I hear this before?" the narrative will genuinely be news to him.

In his aloof detachment, *Lycopodium* might be said to resemble the moon, which sheds light but gives no real warmth. This is especially felt in marriages, in which *Lycopodium* often goes through the correct gestures of love and affection without the strong underlying feelings. Spouses complain of the essential coolness of their *Lycopodium* mates, employing phrases like, "He pretends to care but doesn't really"; "He's never there when I need him emotionally"; "He has no deep feeling for me—or for anybody, it seems. I sometimes wonder if he knows what love is." This last is not necessarily an accurate assessment, but *Lycopodium*'s way of always holding something in reserve, of never giving himself entirely, understandably produces this impression.

The *Lycopodium* male, who thinks well of himself as a husband, is often genuinely surprised by his wife's dissatisfaction. "What's gotten into her? I'm a good provider and a reasonable man, and I believe in marriage. What more does she want?" he asks. To be sure, he is often a steadying influence in a marriage. "Perhaps I'm not all she desires, but I am still her anchor to windward," was one *Lycopodium*'s answer to the complaints of his emotional and excitable spouse. He had a point. His very aloofness provided a ballast that prevented their marriage from capsizing.

However, the most common complaint of the spouse is, "Oh, he is a good enough husband—reliable, pleasant much of the time, or as long as I defer to him. But he seems to like everyone equally, myself included, and I would like to feel I am someone *special* to him." True enough, *Lycopodium* does dislike making distinctions between people, instinctively regarding comparisons as odious. Everyone, he maintains, has both virtues and defects and is therefore more or less on the same plane. He tends to regard people collectively, in a dispassionate way, without seeking to single out certain ones for any particular liking or dislike.

Maybe the reason for *Lycopodium*'s somewhat patronizing "everyone is equal" attitude is that, engrossed in his work and basically satisfied with himself, he has little time or inclination to be interested in others as *individuals*—and particularly in the members of his family as distinct personalities in their own right. He loves them because they are his wife and children, but relates to them less for their own characters and merit than for their relationship to himself. He so takes for granted their love, loyalty, and attention that they begin to sense that he would love a different wife and children just as well.

It is not that *Lycopodium* is ungiving or without emotion. He can be moved by sentiment (as when he is thanked), and he himself feels gratitude. He is a good, dependable friend, and in dealing with him socially or professionally one senses consideration, thoughtfulness, often true kindness. But he cannot tolerate too much closeness and sends out the subconscious signal, "Not too many emotional demands. I like you, but keep your distance." Thus he will not allow others, even those he loves, to penetrate the core of his reserve. And when his inaccessibility or reserve is threatened, it is then that he becomes irritable, critical, sarcastic, caustic, or taciturn.

Lycopodium's need for detachment is fundamental to the careers he chooses and the roles he plays therein. Essentially, he works well within large institutional frameworks—not only because he is attracted to authority and power, but also because by nature he is respectful of institutions as such. They supply a structure for perpetuating the values he so profoundly respects and whose necessity is so apparent to his conservative and practical instincts. This is an important key to the nature. Both intellectually and instinctively he recognizes man's need for institutions to protect hard-won accomplishments and ideals, and he functions well within them because they provide channels through which feelings and impulses are directed in a controlled, contained, and regulated manner.

For *Lycopodium* mistrusts extremes of any kind—intellectual, ideological, emotional, as well as those of taste or personality. Just as he believes that the truth does not lie on any one side but somewhere in between, he likewise is convinced that progress and understanding are possible only by adhering to some middle course.

Because he himself is emotionally low-key and collected he expects others to be the same. Talleyrand voiced the type's instinctive distrust of extreme or emotional behavior when he instructed his colleagues before the diplomatic negotiations at the Congress of Vienna: "Above all, not too much zeal!"

To function effectively, every institution, religious as well as secular, requires in its hierarchies these urbane, socially disposed, politically astute leaders. And those who achieve positions of prominence as chairmen, presidents, elders, and bishops are frequently *Lycopodiums*. Because of this type's understated and courteous manner (the iron hand is well concealed in the velvet glove), mankind on the whole is happy to be led by them. In fact, so skillful at times are these charismatic individuals at establishing and projecting an image of competence and rectitude that if it so happens the Emperor has no clothes, others do not notice.

It was mentioned earlier that *Lycopodium* functions well as diplomat or politician, where his pragmatic instincts and somewhat skeptical manner stand him in good stead. Predictably, his mentality is also well suited for the law, a discipline that supplies his supple mind with scope for intellectual adventure while demanding a certain detachment. Lawyers and especially judges must excel in that which *Lycopodium* does instinctively: weighing, balancing, compromising, moderating, considering the interests of opposing groups and factions, and bending and interpreting facts to achieve viable solutions.

Biographic details of the life of Supreme Court Justice Oliver Wendell Holmes provide an excellent illustration of a predominantly *Lycopodium* mentality. He exhibited *Lycopodium*'s dignified manner, subtle intellect, and sophisticated style; but even his closest friends spoke of his essential coolness and insensitivity in personal relationships. *Lycopodium*-like, Holmes enjoyed socializing and being lionized at the elegant home of Boston Brahmins and prominent Washingtonians, evincing there an almost tireless energy in sophisticated small talk, especially relishing his own repartee and witticisms. When asked by an admiring throng of Boston ladies what he thought of Emile Zola, whose risqué novels were then shocking Puritan New England, Holmes laconically replied, "Improving, but dull." Or, when at the age of eighty he was passed on the street by an attractive young woman, he sighed to his companion, "Oh, to be seventy again!" These bon mots he would then relay to his unfailingly appreciative wife, who usually stayed at home, having neither the strength nor the desire to keep up with his social pace.

Holmes also exhibited the constitutional type's viability in his amazingly productive longevity as a Justice. He sat on the Supreme Court for almost thirty years, a major influence until the day he retired at the age of ninety-one! *Lycopodium,* too, was the ultimate paradox of Holmes' life. His measured and aloof objectivity, judicial fair-mindedness, and intellectual balance prompted him to devote a large part of his long career to upholding the principles of American mass democracy, of which he personally (an elitist by nature and upbringing) strongly disapproved.

Combining duty and dignity, sense of service and feeling for style (his book *The Common Law* is one of the finest examples of legal writing in the English language), humanitarian concern and personal coolness and detachment, Holmes is a splendid representative of the *Lycopodium* nature.

But even the strongest of *Lycopodiums* may have an Achilles' heel, and self-deception is one natural outgrowth of the type's self-esteem, viability, and detachment. To preserve these three, the individual ignores or conceals from himself undesirable realities, refusing even to admit their existence. This attitude of willful blindness was exemplified in the behavior of Lord Horatio Nelson, who, while a captain during the Baltic campaign, when signaled by the admiral's flagship not to engage the enemy, put the telescope to his blind eye and complacently declared, "I do not see the order." He then proceeded into battle (and fought on to victory).

From disregarding facts that interfere with his designs, *Lycopodium* may go on to forget what is fact and what is not. His poor memory—or more precisely, his convenient memory—contributes to this, since he has a good memory for whatever reinforces his current policy but seems genuinely to forget whatever does not. In this way, his self-deception is more complex than mere lying or hypocrisy. Because it satisfies some emotional need and supports his viability, *Lycopodium* genuinely believes that whatever brings him advantage is good and true, whereas everything disagreeable or distasteful must be wrong and untrue.

This trait of accepting only as much reality as he can assimilate without threat to his detachment or his desires is unquestionably an invaluable asset in life. The defect of this virtue, however, is obvious. As mentioned earlier, *Lycopodium* patches up difficulties in relationships instead of confronting them on a deeper level. In the same way he is less willing than perhaps any other constitutional type to acknowledge unacceptable truths about his character, lifestyle, or attitude. He will agree to undergo family counseling or psychotherapy, only to withdraw just as he is beginning to reach some understanding not congenial to his self-image—some hitherto denied moral, emotional, or intellectual inadequacy: "I do not require counseling. My wife may need it, but *I* don't. Anyway, I'm not interested in discussing our problems any longer."

Furthermore, *Lycopodium*'s self-deception allows him to be more easily deceived by others. Although shrewd and full of political savvy, *Lycopodium* can be credulous, deluded by appearances and exhibiting surprisingly poor judgment of people. He is taken in by name-dropping, boasting, flattery, and self-promotion and is impressed by famous or financially successful personages per se. Conversely, he may overlook true worth in a modest individual. But even his poor judgment may work ultimately to his own advantage: the person who is all glitter may be less worthy than *Lycopodium* thinks he is, but may still serve his immediate needs better than one who is true gold.

Thus, *Lycopodium* is often wedded to his self-deception for the simple reason that he does not want to change; and maybe there is no need to change. He is pleased with himself, successful by worldly standards, and wants to remain as he is: self-deceptive on certain subjects, but an effective and viable member of society. After all, a pleasing self-deception involves far less suffering than a sometimes devastating self-knowledge—and is certainly more conducive to productivity. It is the unity of a nature able to filter out the troublesome aspects of life that makes him viable, equipping him perfectly for his worldly tasks. As with moss itself, little modification is needed for survival.

Sometimes, however, *Lycopodium* will display a sincere desire not to remain the unchanging moss, but to grow and to develop in understanding. This trait emerges particularly in the middle years, when his natural unity begins to break down (at which time he begins to be afflicted with one or more of the variety of genitourinary complaints or digestive disorders prominent in this type). He may then lose confidence in his own power and vigor; or, sensing a discrepancy between the public image and the private person behind it, he becomes beset with doubts. "I feel that the rug I've been standing on so securely my whole life has been pulled out from under me," is a characteristic remark. Or, he may say, "Apparently, the foundation on which I built my reputation was never solid. The whole structure of my beliefs has suddenly collapsed." Or, "I don't know what happened, but suddenly my confidence is totally shattered. Is my profession all there is to me?"

It is at this point that the potentized clubmoss can come wonderfully to his aid. He can then, with the customary energy and intelligence of his type, set about making his appearance of heightened vigor, intellectual strength, confidence, and serenity become—or remain—a reality.

Lycopodium

PRINCIPAL REGIONS AFFECTED

Head	Pressing headache from not eating regularly; premature baldness and graying of hair
Throat	Inflammations; infections, especially right-sided
Chest	Various types of **coughs** in both acute and chronic lung conditions
Digestion	**Faulty digestion** with liver and gallbladder dysfunction; feels full and bloated after eating even small amounts of food or, conversely, appetite increases with eating; drowsy after meals; **much flatulence**; colic
Urination	**Slow in coming, must strain**; pain in back before urinating; red sediment in urine; tendency to formation of kidney stones
Male	Prostate enlargement; **decreased sexual impulse**; impotence, especially with wife
Female	Vaginal dryness; painful intercourse; excessive bleeding around menopause; **right ovarian pain**

GENERALITIES

Mental powers remain strong even when physical energy is failing; but also a useful remedy when memory starts failing or the individual starts misusing or misspelling words

Receding hairline or early balding in men; early graying of hair in men and women

Lined face; especially deep furrows in the prominent brow

Right-sided complaints, or moving from right to left

MODALITIES (< worse; > better)

Time	< 4:00 to 8:00 PM
Temperature	< Heat of room, of bed; wind and drafts
	> Cool air and applications; but warm food and drink
Food/Drink	< Legumes, farinaceous food, cabbage family (all cause flatulence)
	> Warm or hot drinks
	Craves sweets and carbohydrates
Other	< Pressure or tightness of clothes, especially around the waist and abdomen

GUIDING MENTAL SYMPTOMS

Highly represented in males of strong intellect—lawyers, politicians, physicians, scholars—who exhibit well-developed diplomatic and leadership skills

Extremely conscious of public and professional image

Respectful of authority, authority figures, and institutions; often achieves positions of power and prestige

Arrogance; intolerant of contradiction or of being thwarted; little things annoy

Self-deception in an otherwise strong mentality

Emotional aloofness; wants people around him, but not too close (preferably in the next room)

Conservative mentality; wariness of undertaking new ventures in personal (not professional) life

Midlife crisis in men, with loss of self-confidence, after having been headstrong, arrogant, and self-willed in earlier life

Anticipatory anxieties before performing in public; fear of breaking down under stress, but possesses the ability to put up a strong front to hide his insecurities

Sepia

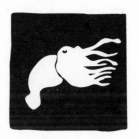

Sepia is made from the fresh ink of the cuttlefish—an independent creature that swims alone rather than in a group and lives in the crevices of rocks in the cool depths of the sea. When in danger, it sends out clouds of ink to cover its escape, and when securing its prey, it ejects the ink as camouflage. Thus, the brownish-black liquid serves both defensive and aggressive purposes. The image of the cuttlefish will, in a number of ways, help us better to understand the complex *Sepia* nature.

The remedy is predominantly female. There are two distinct *Sepia* types: the overworked, exhausted housewife and the woman who flourishes in the world of business and the arts and invests her energies in the workplace. The woman who suffers from backache, headache, and an overall dragged-down feeling exemplifies the first and more traditional picture. No food appeals to her, the very smell of it nauseates, and she wants nothing to do with the rituals of feeding herself or her family. She is so worn out with the cares of home and children that she wants only to lie down and rest; her very eyelids droop from weakness. In her exhaustion she feels stupid, dull, forgetful; and when overwrought, she feels she must hold tightly onto something to prevent herself from screaming. At times, driven to an extreme of irritability, she lashes out at her children and especially her husband. From these characteristics arises the classic picture of the dissatisfied, rebellious woman who wants to leave her husband and children and get away from it all—or she has simply become indifferent to her loved ones. Additionally, the single mother who feels trapped, resenting her role and having no life partner with whom to share her responsibilities, is often a *Sepia*.

Although in certain cases *Sepia* can certainly be found lacking in maternal or wifely instincts, she is not intrinsically devoid of emotion. Feelings run strong and deep in this type, but she is too tired to feel anything except the need to get through the day's work and survive to the next. She simply has no physical or emotional energy left for love. All manifestations of love—marital, parental, and filial, as well as that of close friendship—are a drain on her reserves of energy and an obstacle to her need for privacy and independence. The cuttlefish, after all, is a solitary creature.

Even when not lacking in maternal instincts, *Sepia* does not take readily to motherhood. The role of constantly caring for others' emotional needs is too binding, too physically and psychologically depleting for her constitution, with its interminable female complaints. Indeed, the cuttlefish remedy is prescribed for menstrual complaints of all kinds, including the various disturbances of menopause, and is often called for in disorders of pregnancy as well as for severe postpartum depression and ailments of childbed or nursing. It is also effective in uterine displacements and disorders such as prolapse, "bearing-down" sensations, and fibroids. Perhaps most dramatic of all is its power to counteract female sterility. There have been many babies whose existence the mother attributes to this homoeopathic remedy.

Sepia's immediate family, then, being the greatest emotional drain, is naturally the greatest threat. She may see her husband and children in direct conflict with her need for self-expression, stifling the growth of her individuality. Whereas another type may view them and their love as enhancing her overall development, *Sepia* feels them to be a hindrance—and all too often experiences familial love as merely a responsibility, a confinement, or even a burden.

Yet, even if she is at the end of her resources—even while re-senting her incarceration and struggling against the emotional bonds that confine her to her home, she is restrained from escaping her domestic obligations by her strong sense of duty and a just pride. "These people love me," she reasons. "They expect something of me. Hard as it is, I must live up to their expectations and not disap-point them. I've got to do well as wife, mother, sister, or daughter." Although she needs independence and may want to throw off the burden of imposed love, still, from a sense of the fitness of things, she will put much care into a task that is uncongenial to her nature. She will discharge her family obligations and household duties scrupulously, trying to do it the "right" way. This characteristic is im-portant, since it explains why, contrary to expectation, *Sepia* fre-quently makes a good, even an excellent mother and will raise chil-dren who are contented, attractive, and a pleasure to be around. This is partly because she is not overly protective, sentimental, or permissive; on the contrary, she is often matter-of-fact and stands no nonsense. She does not oppress her children, nor does she attempt to mold them according to some preconceived image—least of all model them on herself. It is hard enough for her to live with one *Sepia,* let alone encourage her offspring along similar lines. She re-spects the child's personality and lets him be himself—yet without overindulgence.

At times *Sepia*'s pride takes the form of lofty reserve. She does not lightly reveal her emotions, preferring to keep her feelings to herself and discouraging any intrusion. She might high-handedly spurn those proffering assistance and does not want to be beholden to anyone. Nor does she want sympathy or to be in any way touched or approached. In fact, she feels resentful at needing help. She has always managed on her own and wants to continue doing so. Therefore, she might appear ungrateful or unresponsive. But of-ten it is her manner that is at fault rather than her heart, for she is basically considerate and has good will. She will offer assistance to those in need, less enthusiastically than some, perhaps, but more re-liably, cooperating in a direct, businesslike way. Thus, to an outsider she gives the impression of having just stepped out of her personal cares and self-absorption to meet another's needs, and the moment she has done her duty by mankind, she will return to her former self-preoccupied state.

When under the stress of daily living, *Sepia* has two ways of reacting: withdrawing or lashing out. Like the cuttlefish, whose ink serves as a screen behind which to hide, *Sepia* may retire into a dark moodiness, deliberately cutting herself off from others. She is unsociable partly because of the physical effort that sociability demands. As one individual said, "I don't even have the strength to comb my hair before going out, to raise my fork to eat or to pull the muscles of my mouth into a smile." She is too fatigued to delight in music, museums, nature, or any form of company. Uninterested in what others are saying, reluctant to contribute anything herself, too tired to follow the conversation (unable to respond or react), she truly feels indifferent to others at the moment and only wants to crawl into her lair and be left alone. However, it is significant that once *Sepia does* make the supreme effort and attends a social gathering—once the adrenaline starts flowing, counteracting her sluggish state—she comes alive, is good company, and enjoys herself thoroughly.

Sepia women claim to be invigorated by energetic motion or physical activity: jogging, cycling, tennis, aerobic exercise, swimming—anything physically bracing, in preference to a quiet stroll in the park or weeding the garden ("I feel so much better after a really good workout!"). Similar to the cuttlefish, whose limbs or tentacles are always in motion in the water, *Sepia* is more comfortable from moving about and worse from any fixed or "locked" position, such as kneeling in church, standing for any length of time, bending over to do the wash (hence *Sepia* used to be known as the "washerwoman's remedy"), or even sitting. Perhaps for the same reason (that is, amelioration from stimulation), she feels exhilarated by thunderstorms.

On the other hand, just as the cuttlefish's ink also serves as a weapon of attack, so in her misery *Sepia* may sporadically lash out at those nearest her. No one can spread darkness and gloom around herself like the discontented *Sepia*. At such times everyone around her must tread cautiously for fear of provoking an angry outburst.

The cuttlefish, however, is not a truly aggressive animal, and *Sepia,* faced with real opposition or a threat, is apt to collapse suddenly and become spineless. She becomes incapable of making decisions and is full of tears and, above all, complaints. No matter how exhausted, she is seldom too tired to complain. Concentrating on the dark side of things, she is convinced that she has a raw deal in life and that fate is against her. Futilely, she may envy one friend her job, another her nicer home, a third her more interesting husband, a fourth her apparent lack of problems. She even envies her own husband's satisfaction at his work. She feels that he is growing and his mind is expanding while she, tied to the home, is contracting and her mind is deteriorating, with no sense of fulfillment. One woman will say drearily, "There is no joy in my life, and, if there were, I would be incapable of appreciating it." Another will complain, "I can't seem to get what I want from life. Is this all there is to it? Do I even have a *right* to a meaningful existence?" A third may lament, "Why can't I be happy as others are? I wish I knew what a normally happy life is!" So pervasive is the black cloud surrounding her that not only is she indifferent to pleasure, but she cannot even envisage the possibility of change or improvement in her life.

Thus, the aura that emanates most strongly from the dissatisfied *Sepia* woman, especially the homemaker, is one of stasis or stagnation. Just as she feels as if nothing is moving in her body (that her digestion and circulation are stagnant, with heavy, weary, dragging-down sensations in various parts), so nothing is moving in her life. She is stuck in a state of weariness, misery, and gloom.

From the housewife seeking emancipation from her too-limited role in the home as spouse and mother, we proceed to the second face of *Sepia*. This is a woman who thrives on the intellectual challenge of a career or profession—finding her niche in a world comparatively devoid of personal emotions. If married and childless, the career woman might say, "I'm quite certain that I don't want to have children. My maternal instinct isn't highly developed; I'm perfectly content with my husband." And she is. She is also generally an admirable and supportive wife, interesting herself in her husband's work, helping him with her good advice and clear intellect, ready to care for him—as long as he does not curtail her independence. Or, if single and asked whether she misses marriage, she might reply, "No, I'm perfectly content with my career and my friends"; or "I miss a good, strong ongoing relationship with a man, but not marriage. I don't want to be tied down, cleaning up after a husband or preparing his meals. I need my own space to get down to my painting and sketching, and I'm happier in a freer relationship." Thus, she is not necessarily antipathetic to sexual relations per se, as the traditional picture of *Sepia* suggests. This picture probably arose because, until recently, sex for women was associated with marriage, housework, and childbirth.

Sepia in her proper element, functioning in the larger world (and this includes the woman who has found a way to exercise her particular talent from her home), is a spirited, creative, contented woman—the possessor of a keen intelligence and a penetrating mind, which helps her excel in traditionally male fields, such as politics, law, and business. Her whole lifestyle might exhibit a striving for independence and self-realization. The type is encountered in such pioneer feminists as Lucy Stone Blackwell and Susan B. Anthony—the feisty, articulate, dedicated, and courageous leaders of the American Women's Suffrage Movement, who, together with their numerous disciples in the nineteenth and twentieth centuries, have valiantly fought for women's equal rights, education, and opportunities in the workplace.

Frequently, *Sepia* is artistic. She dresses stylishly and in good taste and has a good eye for interior decorating. In the creative arts, she often takes up the visual arts: drawing, painting, graphic design. And of all performing arts she prefers dance. In fact, dancing is often a passion with her—possibly because in this form of graceful yet vigorous exercise (reminiscent of the motion of the tentacles of the cuttlefish) she feels free and unconstrained and finds a creative out-let for her pent-up emotions. There was doubtless much *Sepia* in the genius of Isadora Duncan and Martha Graham, founders of schools of modern dance, with their attempts to liberate dance from the too-rigid forms of classical ballet and in their search for new ways for the body to express its inner emotions through movement.

Sepia is also the possessor of a sound and emotionally unbiased judgment, which she is apt to express in a straightforward manner. There is little subterfuge or evasiveness in her nature; in fact, she can even be too outspoken. Being clever, objective, and generally right, she may feel free to point out to others their shortcomings in a rather blunt manner. She might greet an old friend with a hearty, "My, you *have* put on weight!" or "What are you doing with yourself these days, Ellie? Still nothing, as usual? Just hanging around, wasting your time?" Or, a *Sepia* guest might thank her hostess at the end of a din-ner party: "Many thanks for a nice evening. It was lovely seeing you and your husband again, even though this party was not as good as the one I came to last year. Your friends are not as interesting as they used to be." Still, in a curious way, *Sepia* is not usually offensive—and certainly, she is seldom malicious. Rather, she is candid and di-rect, stating facts that cannot be disputed in the dispassionate tones of a weather forecaster announcing that today's temperature is eighty-six degrees, with a thirty percent chance of rain.

Moreover (and this is a rare quality), *Sepia* displays a funda-mental *self*-honesty. If she is direct in her manner toward others, she is equally forthright about herself. She understands her own nature and is aware of her weaknesses as well as her strengths. Part of her seeming indifference or lack of feeling originates in this dispassion-ate self-judgment. Thus, a woman undergoing a traumatic divorce might say, "Of course I am sad to see my twenty-five year marriage dissolve. I love my husband, and this is entirely his decision. But maybe I helped undermine the relationship by telling him he really didn't love me—or that if he knew me better he wouldn't. I know I have a perverse tendency to undermine close relationships; I don't know why." And from a sense of pride, she may attempt to preserve a strong front by adding, "On the other hand, it seems that women grow more through disappointment in love than through any other experience. So [with a shrug that dispels undue emotionalism or self-pity], why should I be exempt from this opportunity for growth?"

In an attempt to be candid about herself, however, *Sepia* might tend to put herself down: "I'm not good enough at what I'm doing. . . . Nobody really needs me at work . . . and I don't think they really like me. . . . I feel like I'm a burden to others—a real drag. . . ." Or a generous *Sepia* woman may consider herself ungenerous (even while she puts out more emotional and physical energy into helping another than is her natural inclination) because she lacks *spontaneous* generosity.

Sepia herself might be reluctant to acknowledge her virtues, but others, on closer acquaintance, learn to value her for her good qualities: fairness, candor, trustworthiness, self-honesty—and perhaps most important of all, integrity. One knows where she stands on important issues and knows that she will abide by her convictions.

Among literary heroines it is Scarlett O'Hara in *Gone With the Wind* who vividly exhibits several characteristics of this second face of *Sepia*. With her sharp business mind and constant striving for independence and self-expression, she seeks to emancipate herself from the "female" virtues of pliancy, docility, gentleness, and submissiveness so assiduously cultivated in the antebellum South. Characteristic, too, are her passion for dancing and her forthright speech and conduct (which give rise to so much public censure), as well as her admirable (even if reluctant) loyalty and responsibility toward her family—a long and heavy burden on her. Finally, *Sepia*-like is Scarlett's courage, born of pride, in the face of trying circumstances, as she struggles to survive the ravages of the Civil War and the Reconstruction and a series of heavy personal losses. As one character in the novel says of her, "I like the way you meet things . . . even if they are disagreeable. You take your fences cleanly, like a good hunter."

Although *Sepia* is encountered far less frequently in males than in females, the remedy was originally discovered by Hahnemann in a male patient: a painter displaying unusual symptoms, whom Hahnemann observed inadvertently poisoning himself by constantly licking the tip of his brush while painting in sepia ink (in this way "proving" the remedy*).

The male mental symptoms are at times a curious counterpart to the female ones. The woman seeks to emancipate herself from the passive, receptive female role, the world of home and emotions, and enter into a life of action. The male, conversely, weary of the competitive struggle, wants to disengage from the active world of politics and business and heavy responsibilities in order to lead a quieter, more contemplative life. The formerly energetic, hard-working man, now middle-aged or elderly, is discontented with his job and tired or worn out emotionally. He wants to retire to the peace and quiet of the country, there to pursue some low-keyed occupation or hobby—or simply be left alone. Yet he too is better from strenuous activity: chopping wood, spading the garden, brisk five-mile walks.

One woman's lament about her intellectual husband's recently changed behavior provides an example of the male *Sepia*. "He has always had a first-rate mind [she observed], but recently, instead of being interested in anything significant, all he talks about is the high price and poor quality of groceries. Also, he complains if there is a bit of unused food left lying in the refrigerator. When he comes home from work, even as he turns the key in the lock, he can smell something aging in the refrigerator. Then he fishes it out and dangles it in front of my nose and says, '*What's this?*' Or he nags if I use the wrong kitchen utensils to cook with. He just hangs around me being picky and petty over everything and chronically dissatisfied." The woman also recalled another incident illustrating her husband's *Sepia*-blunt behavior. At the conclusion of a lecture they had attended the husband approached the speaker and asked, "Are you

---

*See the *Introduction* for more information.

sure you are the same person whose picture is on the back of your books? I would never have recognized you! You've certainly aged since that photograph—and where is your hair?"

Noteworthy, however, is that similar to the woman, the *Sepia* man will exhibit a rare self-honesty. He does not harbor a higher than warranted idea of his own capacities, and is capable of judging himself, like others, dispassionately and with penetration.

Every person is composed of both male and female characteristics. Generally, the conscious personality has the attributes of the physically expressed gender, while the unconscious bears marks of the opposite gender and performs a complementary balancing function. In the *Sepia* type, characteristics of the other gender surface in a way in which the individual must consciously understand and direct; otherwise, they take on a dark or oppressive nature. *Sepia*'s challenge, then, is to creatively express the unconscious gender— thereby moving out of chronic dissatisfaction or gloom (the deep, dark waters in which the cuttlefish makes its home) into the bracing daylight.

Sepia

PRINCIPAL REGIONS AFFECTED

Head	**Pains in terrible shocks (usually left-sided)**; frequently with nausea, vomiting
Digestion	**Empty feeling in stomach, not relieved by eating;** burning pains, abdominal bloating; **nausea from sight, smell, or even thought of food; constipation**
Female	**Chronic cystitis;** involuntary urination when coughing, laughing, or sneezing; yellowish, greenish vaginal discharges with much itching; vaginal dryness, painful intercourse, absence of or little sexual desire
	Numerous menstrual complaints: premenstrual symptoms, headache, cramping, nausea and vomiting, backache; excessive bleeding or absent menses; intramenstrual bleeding or spotting; **menopausal hot flashes, palpitations, tremulous feeling;** uterine prolapse, easy dislocation of pelvis; "bearing-down" sensation of pelvic organs; infertility
	Complaints of pregnancy and childbirth: morning sickness, abnormal food cravings, lower back pain; tendency to miscarry; complaints after miscarriage or abortion; postpartum depression ("baby blues")
Back	**Weakness and/or pain in small of back;** better lying on something hard or from firm support; pains extend to back
Skin	Various discolorations and eruptions: circumscribed red or brown spots (ringworm), **adult acne, pimply eruptions along margin of hair;** herpetic eruptions around mouth and nose; cracks on lower lip; eczema

GENERALITIES

Predominantly a female remedy

Overall weariness and weakness

Emotional state of stasis is reflected in the physical feelings of sluggishness or stagnation

Bearing-down sensation or dragged-down feeling of parts affected

Pains shoot upward

Sensation of a ball or lump in inner parts (stomach, uterus, bladder, rectum)

Generally left-sided complaints

Continued.

Sepia—*cont'd*

MODALITIES (< worse; > better)

Time < Morning and evening; **monthly**

Temperature < Cold wind, dampness; **before thunderstorms**

> Cold bathing (especially of affected parts); warmth of bed, hot applications

> During and after thunderstorms

Position < **Locked position:** sitting (must cross limbs); kneeling, standing; lying on left side

> **Lying down**

Energy > Regular exercise; **vigorous motion (especially dancing);** sleep, even if only a short nap

Food/Drink < Milk

> Desire for vinegar, pickles, tart, sour, or acid foods

GUIDING MENTAL SYMPTOMS

Picture of the exhausted, overworked housewife seeking to escape her responsibilities, but seeing no way out

Stifled emotions; indifferent to loved ones

Irritability, anger at contradiction

Woman of artistic bent working in the visual arts or writing

The contented, capable career woman

Clever, straightforward, perceptive

Middle-aged men and women who are discontented with their lives and are searching for more gratification

Fear of solitude (even if averse to company), illness, poverty; anxiety over trifles

Sulphur

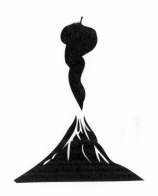

Even as the element sulphur is generously diffused throughout the earth's crust beneath the surface vegetation (as we know from the various sulphuric gases and ejecta of volcanic exhalations), so a *Sulphur* layer lies beneath the surface of virtually every human being. This is observed in the way a *Sulphur* picture emerges during the different stages of life in constitutional types other than its own: in diseases of infancy and childhood, complaints of adolescence, midlife crises in men, menopausal ailments in women, and in the weaknesses and infirmities of old age.

Likewise, this remedy is called upon repeatedly during the various stages of acute or chronic illness in any sufferer. Because of its well-attested power to bring latent symptoms to the surface, *Sulphur* is often the first remedy used in a severe chronic disease; here, in its opening role, it might actually jump the claim of a seemingly more "similar" remedy and single-handedly resolves the entire malady. It is equally effective in the middle of a course of treatment when, other medicines failing, it displays a unique capacity to elicit a response—either in itself prodding stagnant cases into progress or by activating the previously ineffective well-selected remedy. Finally, *Sulphur* frequently plays an Omega as well as an Alpha role in illnesses or ailments by hastening convalescence and cure during their subsiding stage—as well as by being invaluable in the treatment of conditions that tend to relapse.

In seeking further correspondences between the medicinal substance and human constitutional types, we recall that elemental sulphur is well known as a powerful external and internal cleansing agent—hence the use of sulphur baths, soaps, and drinking waters. Similarly, every person can, at some point in his life, benefit from this protean remedy's capacity to clean out a host of accumulated toxins, impurities, or residual ailments—as well as the undesirable side effects of traditional Western medications.

Sulphur's wide range of activity does not, however, preclude its possessing a personality distinctly its own. In former times sulphur was called *brimstone,* from the Middle English words for "burning stone," and the element has long been used for such purposes as the manufacture of matches and gunpowder. This image, together with that of the volcano, yields the characteristics of burning, eruptiveness, and flare-up, and indeed, the *Sulphur* individual easily becomes heated. On the physical level, he perspires freely and profusely, cannot tolerate the heat of a room or of his bed, opens windows to let in cold air, and throws off extra clothes by day or his blankets at night. Many of his internal complaints and general symptoms have a burning quality to them. He is also prone to numerous skin eruptions of the heated, red, itching variety. As with a volcano, the remedy's action is centrifugal (pushing from within outward), so that *Sulphur*'s disturbed energy often manifests through skin conditions.

Sulphur's heat-emitting temperament emerges early in life in the boisterous youngster and continues throughout adolescence. And even though after adolescence the heat of the personality subsides somewhat, the young adult often remains feisty and assertive, ceaselessly on the go. The onset of middle age might well generate an increase or resumption of emotional heat. The male, especially, grows critical and belligerent, prone to raise his voice when irritated, even if only over minutiae. His temper flares easily and his outbursts are strong—like a volcano that blows its top and spews forth sulphur. But also like a volcano, which once the internal pressure has been released is quiet again, *Sulphur,* who is quick to erupt, is equally quick to subside. Minutes after his outburst he has already forgotten his anger and the reason for it. Moreover, in certain cases, violent flare-ups occur, but rarely. One woman stated that when her *Sulphur* future husband proposed, she had hesitated because of his explosive temper. "Don't worry about that, my dear," he assured her. "Vesuvius is quiet most of the time." And this proved to be an accurate self-characterization.

The type is often argumentative, finding in verbal combat an outlet for his heat and pugnacity. It is often a *Sulphur* who fires off the first shot. Since he enjoys an argument for its own sake, both as a form of mental exercise and as an exchange of ideas, he is not particular about the topic chosen for this purpose and is ever ready to jump in with both feet into any chance battle (like the Irishman in the anecdote who, seeing two men pummeling each other in a bar, inquires: "Is this a private fight, or can anyone join in?"). Furthermore, because his arguments remain largely on the intellectual plane, his feelings are rarely deeply affected. His love of contention overcomes any wound, and he looks forward with pleasurable excitement to the next verbal confrontation—and his probable triumph. For with his tendency to wear down an opponent, he is difficult to best in an argument.

Another facet of *Sulphur*'s heated temperament is a strong need for personal recognition. Whatever is going on around him, he must be at the center of the action—"the bride at every wedding and the corpse at every funeral" (as was said of Teddy Roosevelt). He is the classic entrepreneur. He might also be the person who boasts loudly and at length of his numerous accomplishments, innovative ideas, or future plans; or he vaunts his correct political or financial predictions (which may be only hindsight). At times he succeeds in building a reputation not only on what he has already accomplished but also on what he *intends* to do. His conversational egocentrism is caricatured in the account of two men talking. When the first has finished a long monologue, he turns to his companion and says, "But enough about me—let's talk about you. Tell me, what do you think of my latest book?"

Finally, due to an inherently optimistic mentality, many a *Sulphur* is constitutionally unable to see faults in any of his personal actions or in whatever belongs to him—just as he cannot see any defects in any of his schemes or ventures (thinking, "If it's mine, it must be admirable"). Generally speaking, this person of large ideas has a need to make everything under his patronage worthy of his interest and as large as himself.

The range of action of *Sulphur,* the remedy, is so broad that its personality picture is bound to display variants, shadow-sides, and opposites, and therefore is best approached in the light of its polarities.

One of the type's most prominent polarities is selfishness and generosity. Self-absorption renders him oblivious to the needs of others; and an extreme form of selfishness is encountered in the blatant egoist who is so completely engrossed in his own world that he will not put himself out for anyone. He strongly approves of people helping each other out in life, provided this is not expected of him. Indeed, everything is owed him ("What's mine is mine, and what's yours is negotiable"). In his lack of consideration for others he is convinced that nothing is difficult, fatiguing, or important to anyone but himself, and he will come home to a wife laden with household cares and small children and grumble, "Why didn't you rake up the leaves as I asked you to do? What do you mean you didn't have time? What *have* you been doing all day?" Nor is this churlish behavior limited to the home. Lost in his great thoughts of saving the world or building a fortune, he has no time to cooperate in some communal enterprise, or pull his share. Not only does he expect others to look after his comforts, but he actually expects them to feel privileged to do so.

At times, however, the complete reverse is encountered. Instead of being selfish, *Sulphur* is the soul of generosity, overflowing with benevolence. He is the warm-hearted man (or woman) who will not turn away any personal demand on his purse and who is constantly being approached for the expenditure of time and energy on some charitable cause. He can be exceptionally hospitable; the act of throwing a party gives him immense satisfaction. He likes to entertain on a lavish scale, throwing open the doors to all and sundry— the more the merrier. Like an enthusiastic but inexperienced cook, he insists on throwing the most incompatible ingredients (incongruous personalities) into a common pot (social venture), sanguine that a delicious dish will result (a good time will be had by all). Although the odds may seem heavily against him, his concoctions often succeed—seasoned as they are with his own abundant energy and good spirits, which pull others along in their wake. Similarly, in the workplace, a *Sulphur* will throw together the most disparate business associates to make a successful venture. Or he may invite one and all to participate in some epic enterprise initiated by himself.

Characteristically, though, each one of his generous impulses must still somehow redound to his own credit—for *Sulphur* seeks recognition even in his munificence. Thus, the guests at his party were "the most interesting and extraordinary group of people I've ever encountered," the wine served had "the most exquisite bouquet of any I've tasted in years," and the food was prepared by "without exception, the most talented chef you will find on the East Coast—a true genius." And in his gift-bestowing propensities, the present of a crate of fresh peppers or tomatoes will be proffered to a friend with the boast, "My vegetable garden is the envy of the neighborhood. All my neighbors are in agreement that this year's crop is the *finest* I've ever produced!" So high a premium does *Sulphur* place on the quality of giving (every bit as high as on the blessedness of receiving) that in his eyes, generosity is the seal of his righteousness. Certainly, no other type enjoys contemplating this particular virtue more than he. And since he habitually paints on a large canvas, fortunately for him, he has an almost inexhaustible subject for contemplation.

At times *Sulphur* can be too generous for his own or another's good, behaving in a mistakenly liberal manner. He willingly supports brothers-in-law and other family members, or friends who are loafers and hangers-on, repeatedly bailing them out financially and otherwise, to the detriment of their own character development— not to mention the inconvenience or disservice to his own family. Other constitutional types may also be generous, but it is *Sulphur's* irrepressible geniality, together with his universal (not to say indiscriminate) kindness, that make him a strikingly benevolent figure.

A related polarity is *Sulphur's* materialism and antimaterialism. This personality type innately harbors a strong materialistic streak, the most obvious manifestation of which is his attitude toward money. The wealthy individual characteristically spends his money extravagantly and ostentatiously: on expensive cars, stereos, over-sized mansions, and other status symbols. (One *Sulphur* described himself as "heavily into conspicuous consumption.") Whether he is well off or not, money is a subject of which he never wearies. He is fascinated by the price of things and by how much money others are earning—and these subjects constitute the nonintellectual type's principal themes of conversation. Moreover, even if affluent, he will talk just as happily about the high price of string beans or soda water.

The majority of *Sulphurs* exhibit a sound financial sense, whether they are running a small grocery store, managing a large corporation, or dealing in shares, stocks, and bonds. Many of these individuals appear to have as their sole life's goal the wresting of a fortune from compliant or defiant opportunity. Money, during these earning power years, becomes the principal measure of personal worth, and the type judges another's talents and capacities by how much money he earns or is capable of earning. Later in life he might enjoy donating the wealth that he has accumulated to large, prestigious institutions, or he may establish his own charitable foundation and see to it that he is given credit for his largesse. He thus satisfies his generous as well as acquisitive instincts and succeeds in serving both God and Mammon.

On the other hand, some *Sulphurs* are tight-fisted, disliking to lend money or to spend it on others or even on themselves. Such is the husband who complicates his family's life by insisting on unnecessary petty economies. He sets the home thermostat uncomfortably low, refuses to buy a kettle with a whistle that works, and drives a car that is a wreck. He loves economy for its own sake, although each individual has his own particular quirk. For instance, a successful writer will type his manuscripts on the reverse sides of letters, bills, and other scraps of paper that most people would throw away or recycle. This is the kind of economy *Sulphur,* who abhors waste, cannot resist. He enjoys nothing more than making dinner out of leftovers or salvaging a "perfectly good" piece of wire from a dismantled dishwasher to repair the electrical system of his car. In fact, he will hoard just about anything he can lay his hands on. A packrat by nature, he hates to part with any object, even the most useless, and is constitutionally unable to throw things away, because "Who knows? Some day it might come in handy."

Furthermore, however cluttered his office, basement, or room, he dislikes anything to be out of sight or reach, and cannot bear having anything moved or removed. The *Sulphur* desk is easily recognized by the books and papers heaped up or scattered around, so that it would appear impossible to find anything. Yet he can in a moment locate the smallest memorandum and is distraught if anyone suggests removing some papers and putting things in order. He himself regards clutter and messy surroundings as "comfort."

Simultaneously, *Sulphur* might possess a theoretical desire for neatness. Becoming upset by the ambient dirt and mess, he will make a Herculean effort to pick up after himself. But the apparent neatness of his abode is purely superficial, and disorder reigns beneath the surface order. If a closet door is opened, all the contents—hastily pushed out of sight—will come tumbling out, and his desk drawers are a rat's nest, with pencils, pens, rubber-bands, string, and paper clips entangled in an inextricable bundle.

Sulphur's materialism evinces itself in yet another related way: he is the quintessential collector—of stamps, books, records, work tools, matchboxes, ashtrays; you name it. The financially successful person satisfies his collector's instincts by acquiring *objets d'art,* with which he will fill his house to bursting point. Extremely pleased with and proud of his collection, he talks of it, displays it, and is not even envious of a rival's possessions—although naturally, he would always like to add to his own.

Conversely, *Sulphur* might demonstrate a total absence of interest in material things or financial matters. With his head in the clouds, he is so engrossed in elevated thoughts that the material world passes by him unobserved. This type will be examined in greater detail below. Suffice it to say that total indifference to material possessions may reflect the type's unworldliness—or it may reflect a conscious principled determination to dispense with the chattels of this world for the sake of spiritual or intellectual development. Like Thoreau living in his one-room cabin at Walden Pond, seeking to return to the simplicity of nature, this *Sulphur* will live ascetically in stark surroundings and, refusing to own anything of value, subsist on the barest minimum.

Even the individual who seeks possessions and enjoys owning them may exhibit a truly antimaterialistic streak in his attitude toward clothes. Thus, the preferred outfit of a well-to-do *Sulphur* might be a twenty-year-old tweed jacket with well-worn elbows or poorly applied patches, which he refuses to part with, and a pair of creased and oversized trousers seemingly acquired from Goodwill. By virtue of being long with him and much worn, his clothes have become true and trusted friends—even more, a part of himself. And how can one throw out a part of oneself?

In concluding this section, one additional aspect of *Sulphur's* particular material bent should be noted: his love of working with his hands and with the soil. This constitutional type is often fascinated by tools and all things mechanical or electrical, evincing from youth a sound grasp of their functioning. Any inventor will have a strong *Sulphur* streak—whether a genius like Thomas Edison or an unknown tinkerer in his cellar who plugs away for years on a solar-powered can opener, a noiseless blender, or a chainless bicycle, until he finally does succeed in discovering something. Likewise, the tenacious small farmer who is content to eke out a bare existence from his plot of land, the hired laborer who enjoys manual work in the garden or yard, the prosperous planter with his expensive machinery and newest technological improvements, and the deskbound businessman who is happiest relaxing in his vegetable patch ("I love my vegetable garden with its turnips and squash. There is nothing in the world I like better than getting my hands *dirty* in the soil")—all are following their *Sulphur* inclinations.

Another prominent *Sulphur* polarity is intellectualism versus antiintellectualism. Whether a farmer or a corporate executive, a blue-collar worker or white-collar one, an artist, scientist, or physician, the intellectual *Sulphur* displays a philosophical slant of mind. He loves rationalizing, theorizing, and weaving abstract or hypothetical systems. Given the opportunity, he will provide a philosophical underpinning for every one of his opinions or in support of some simple action.

From an early age, *Sulphur* enjoys reading instructive works, such as newspapers, science magazines, history books, and encyclopedias—anything to do with the storage and retrieval of statistical data or scientific or historic facts. He may possess a prodigious memory. Once some bit of information lodges in his brain, it stays there accumulating interest, as safely and surely as money in the bank, to be brought out whenever some expenditure is needed. As a conversationalist he will have a vast store of quotations in reserve from writers, classical and popular, ancient and modern—something for every occasion. He remembers complex mathematical formulas, little-known dates in history, and obscure scholarly references. In addition, he might possess an amazing talent for languages. The person who claims to know four or five languages well will invariably have *Sulphur* strong in his constitutional picture. On some level all such intellectual acquisitions can be seen as extensions of the *Sulphur* "collector's" instinct. He accumulates facts and figures, acquires statistical knowledge, and stores information and foreign words as voraciously as he collects worldly goods.

At the same time, *Sulphur* also is the individual who forgets the names of familiar streets, friends, and family members: "You—you— Tom—I mean Tim—whatever your name is . . ." he will say to his son-in-law, Ted, who has been in the family for fifteen years; and he cannot for the life of him recall who came to dinner last week. Or, forgetting a recently held conversation, *Sulphur* (at any mature age) might begin to repeat himself, in exactly the same phrases—not a word changed, not a comma omitted. Such strengths and weaknesses of memory reflect the individual's natural inclination toward the abstract, factual, and scholarly, rather than the purely personal.

Consequently, *Sulphur* is the ragged philosopher: the unkempt, scraggly bearded, unworldly individual of philosophical bent, who lives in a world of ideas and abstractions, where learning and books are as natural to him as breathing. An even more familiar figure is the absent-minded professor, whose mind is so lost in great thoughts that when studying in a library he loses all sense of time and comes home hours late for dinner. Or, if preparing his own meal, he starts reading a book and forgets to turn off the gas under the burning pot. He may be virtually incapable of survival on his own. Far from being the manually dexterous and mechanically adept type discussed earlier, he is impractical and inept with his hands, sometimes unable to drive a car or even to use a typewriter successfully—while opening a can of soup, untying a knotted piece of string, pouring liquid from one bottle into another, let alone fixing a slipped bicycle chain, are all traumatic experiences.

The professorial *Sulphur* can be identified by his manner of presentation. He is well informed on his subject but tends to expostulate on it in too ponderous or exhaustive a fashion. The individual who sometimes appears brilliant, sometimes merely tedious, is probably *Sulphur* (who is a bit of both). He knows so much!—and must be respected for the legitimate scholar or particular authority that he is. Yet, despite the valuable and mind-enriching information pouring out, his style of presentation makes listening difficult. His weakness is the need to communicate *everything* he knows. Listeners soon become glassy-eyed waiting for him to end. Whenever a listener feels like crying out to the speaker, "Stop telling me so much about things I don't want to know!" or "Not *more!*" he can suspect that he is dealing with a *Sulphur.*

Even in everyday conversation *Sulphur* tends to theorize and occasionally to pontificate, and mundane topics take on grand dimensions. He will express himself with as much eloquence on the merits and drawbacks of two different kinds of pens as on the difference between Positivism and Structuralism in contemporary philosophy. Often, too, he expresses himself impersonally, producing on the listener the impression Gladstone did on Queen Victoria—causing her to remark irritably, in one of her rare flashes of wit, "He always addresses me as if I were a public meeting."

Although pedantry, weightiness, and exhaustiveness often characterize *Sulphur*'s presentation of ideas, this does not mean that he is not interesting. On the contrary: like a volcano erupting in all directions, his restless, creative, ever-questing mind is often inventive and original, as he generates theories about both the knowable and the unknowable. Many of the world's strongest and most profound intellects have been *Sulphurs,* who have produced works of universal stature and significance—works that have provided mankind with much of its intellectual dynamism over the centuries.

The *Sulphur* mind takes an encyclopedic approach to the organization of knowledge. Massive compendiums and exhaustive commentaries such as the Talmud (with its unending interpretation and elaboration of the Torah) are *Sulphur* in conception as well as style. Thomas Aquinas' *Summa Theologica,* with its methodical intellectualization of questions of faith and salvation and classification as to who stands where in the eyes of God and the moral order of the universe, embodies the *Sulphur* mind at work. This is also true of Karl Marx's *Das Kapital,* a work that has so profoundly influenced the course of history, yet is so seldom read in its entirety—being far too "*Sulphur*" for ordinary literary consumption. Eighteenth-century author and man of letters Samuel Johnson provides yet another graphic picture. A scholar of remarkable talents, he was reputed to have read more books than any man alive and was a prolific author in many genres: poetry, biography, essays, prayers, meditations, travelogues, aphorisms—not to mention being the author and compiler of the great English Dictionary (lexicography being a highly *Sulphur* occupation).

In a book on homoeopathy, perhaps the most apposite illustration of a *Sulphur* genius is Samuel Hahnemann himself. He had an explosive temper that thrived on controversy and contention and a mind that boldly expounded provocative and controversial medical opinions. He also possessed a phenomenal memory, which enabled him to be a foremost scholar in fields other than the purely medical. He exhibited proficiency in at least five languages beside his native German (French, Italian, English, Latin, and Greek) and, if the hagiography built up around him is to be trusted, competence in several others. He was also the leading chemist of his generation and is considered a not insignificant figure in the history of that discipline. But then, he was an exceedingly fatiguing lecturer. When teaching homoeopathy at the University of Leipzig, he drove most students away by his disorganized material, and poorly presented ideas. Having little patience to organize, in a cogent, systematic manner, truths that were so obvious to him, instead he spent his time showering on his audience invective against traditional Western medicine, heaping it with platitudinous moralizations. Then, too, his *Organon of Medicine,* which needs to be read at least three times for comprehension, illustrates the dense scholarly *Sulphur* style. Most significantly, Hahnemann possessed the *Sulphur* breadth of vision that sparks the great changes and revolutions of the world. Not only, by redefining the concept of "similarity" in therapeutics, did he develop a complete philosophy of medicine, to which nothing essential has needed to be added since its inception (even as it grows in relevance and significance with every passing generation); by discovering a method of "diluting" the medicines and then "proving" them he was able to make his theories practical and accessible to doctors and laymen alike.*

---

*See *Introduction* for further information.

The type's strength in theoretical understanding and need to build systems is not limited, however, to the words of philosophers, writers, healers, and theologians. Johann Sebastian Bach, who, in addition to an almost superhuman output of musical compositions, took upon himself to elaborate and fix for all time the tempered scale for keyboard instruments, and who systematized the principles of functional harmony—thereby establishing the rules of composition for all the subsequent development of classical music—was eminently *Sulphur.*

Indeed, for sheer intellectual vigor, endurance, and productivity, and above all breadth of vision, the *Sulphur* mentality is difficult to surpass. Proceeding from the premise that, within a given discipline, one comprehensive idea or vision can encompass and ultimately define the sum of human experience, the bold mind incorporates large theoretical concepts and vast fields of knowledge into an all-embracing system. This accomplishment, together with the type's pioneering intellectual energy, permits him to contemplate and carry out schemes of a magnitude that others would not consider even possible.

Not all *Sulphur* visionaries, however, are movers and builders. Some are "all talk and no action" dreamers whose impractical or overambitious plans are doomed to remain unrealized. Others embark on an intrinsically worthy scheme, such as raising money for some world-saving mission, learning a Third World language, undertaking to restore a historic building, or translating the works of some obscure Asian poet, but do not follow through. In everyday life this trait comes out in the man who starts but never finishes tasks or repairs around the house—and will not even pick up his tools or the building materials. They lie around waiting for him, while he has already started on another grandiose project. Still other *Sulphurs,* strong in conceptualizing large-scale projects, and even in completing them, are yet weak in attending to the details that lead to real success. One such individual of solid musical ability set himself the goal of memorizing all thirty-two of the Beethoven piano sonatas.

He succeeded in this giant enterprise and was able to plow his way through the entire corpus, but all the sonatas sounded alike.

Sulphur is also recognized in the polar opposite of the energetic, productive type—in the man who is averse to all work and sits around at home all day, reclining in an armchair and thinking his great thoughts. He seeks recognition without feeling any need to exert himself for it; then is disappointed at the world's failure to recognize his genius. Still other *Sulphurs* disdain the education they were fortunate enough to receive, or deny it in favor of some "beyond-learning" mystical or metaphysical philosophy. They begin to feel that they possess a deeper comprehension, which allows them to dispense with the dearly bought core of classical knowledge that is our heritage as human beings. In a word, this constitutional type offers the extremes of overvaluation and undervaluation of formal education.

Above all, even though *Sulphur* may absorb massive amounts of information, his ability to use it appropriately is, at times, deficient. He is knowledgeable enough in the separate components of a discipline but is unable to integrate them. This tendency to miss the forest for the trees leads to a faulty perspective, causing him to be dubbed the "false philosopher," and the lesser *Sulphur* mind can become bogged down in futile, because insoluble, religio-philosophical contemplations, with a penchant for "pondering on the imponderable" (as one *Sulphur* said of himself). For instance, a person might find himself endlessly ruminating on primary causes. And in the Middle Ages, such fruitless conjecturing as "How many angels can dance on the head of a pin?" was a *reductio ad absurdum* of the *Sulphur* speculative mode.

Significantly, however, in a typical *Sulphur* polarity, many fine clerics and eminent theologians (of all religious denominations), true mystics, and teachers or leaders of various spiritual paths will have this remedy prominent in their constitutions.

Last to be mentioned is the direct contrast to *Sulphur*'s robust, creative mentality—namely, his melancholy. Sometimes depression is caused by an overtaxed mind, fatigued by too prolonged or too intense study. The relentless seeker after truth might sit up night after night, devouring books, in his desire to accumulate *all* available knowledge. Then, one day the exhausted mind gives out, leaving him in despair at having lost his most highly developed faculty. The picture of melancholia can also emerge with age when an ossification of the mental faculties takes place and the former broad understanding begins to narrow. At this time of life, too, *Sulphur* may succumb to a religious melancholy. He may be devout, but his view of humanity and human destiny takes on a dark tinge and he finds little comfort in his faith. Or, led astray by his religious searchings and meditations, he succumbs to non-productive anxieties of conscience. But, with the administration of a course of *Sulphur* one can observe the mind and emotions expand, and the elderly individual begins to espouse a happier frame of mind—thus, beautifully exemplifying the homoeopathic conviction that the mind need not contract with age, but that a person ages because his mind contracts.

Sulphur has been discussed primarily as a male remedy, even though women require it as a constitutional medicine almost as frequently as men. But in women the mental characteristics described above are generally more attenuated and subdued—possibly because they are less "pure" types (in the same way as one rarely encounters pure *Sepia* males). The woman is recognized not so much by her eruptive temper (although this certainly can be a feature) as by her high energy, which flourishes when she finds herself surrounded by turmoil and agitation—in an atmosphere that she herself calls "creative disorder." She can simultaneously feed her children, bake bread, carry on a business conversation on the telephone, follow a television program—and in the interim attend to her knitting or paperwork. The same scenario is encountered in the workplace. The more activity and excitement around her, or the more excitement she herself can generate, the more she is stimulated to produce. Additionally, as with the *Sulphur* male, she will come up with a surprisingly well-organized finished product, given the chaos and commotion during the gestation and preparatory periods of any venture.

One example of a predominantly *Sulphur* female intellect is Maria Montessori, the great pioneer in child education, whose visionary mind and profound philosophical grasp of the learning processes of a child's absorbent mind (set forth in a number of long-winded and weighty books, which were to revolutionize all subsequent development in child education) argues for the presence of much *Sulphur* in her constitution. A second historic figure is Mary Baker Eddy, founder of Christian Science—and the only woman in recorded history to found a major world religion. This feat, which she accomplished virtually single-handedly, in the face of much ridicule and opposition, and which called for extraordinary audacity and leadership skills, also financial genius and phenomenal organizational and administrative powers—let alone a breadth of spiritual vision—carries a distinctive *Sulphur* flavor.

All the characteristics examined in this chapter are, however, but drops in the *Sulphur* ocean. The range of symptoms the medicine addresses, its depth of action, and its capacity to act beneficially in all human types at every stage of life (from cradle to grave) renders it far greater than any description of it—far greater than the sum of its parts. Indeed, in its ubiquity and strong polarities, the remedy stands as the highest tribute to the homoeopathic discipline's ability to encompass the wealth and diversity of human nature within a given constitutional type, even while retaining its quintessentially individualizing mode of treatment.

Sulphur

PRINCIPAL REGIONS AFFECTED

Head Heat on top of the head; fullness, pressure; pounding, congestive pains, or sick headache; vertigo; dry, itchy scalp; hair falling out; red orifices: ears, lips, margin of eyelids, inside of nose; bitter taste in the mouth

Digestion Complete loss of or excessive appetite; sudden hunger and weakness (especially around 11:00 AM); acidity, sour eructations, hypoglycemic headaches from skipping meals or delayed eating; diarrhea early in the morning, drives him out of bed; itching and burning in rectum; hemorrhoids

Urination Frequent, urgent need to urinate; passes great quantities of colorless urine, especially at night; burning during urination

Male Stitching pains in genital organs; itching of organs

Female Various menstrual complaints, including premenstrual symptoms; itching and burning of genital organs and discharges; offensive perspiration; menopausal hot flashes, palpitations, vertigo, shortness of breath

Skin Many complaints manifest on the skin; eruptions are red, burning, itching, dry or moist; rough, scaly, unwashed, unhealthy looking skin; adolescent acne, eczema, psoriasis; profuse perspiration

GENERALITIES

Generally warm-blooded, with a tendency to perspire profusely and ebullitions of heat to the head

Uneven distribution of body heat, some parts hot, others cold

Burning, throbbing, congestive nature of many complaints (as of head, chest, stomach, joints, etc.); also redness and inflammation characterize many complaints

Strong (often offensive) odor to perspiration, flatulence, bowel movements, and other discharges

Talks, jerks, and twitches in sleep; wakes up suddenly, with feeling of inability to breathe

Dreams are vivid and action-packed; colorful, exciting, fantastic, absurd; pleasant as well as unpleasant

When other remedies fail, *Sulphur* often stimulates the reactive powers of the organism; also resolves lingering ailments

Continued.

Sulphur—cont'd

MODALITIES (< worse; > better)

Time   < 11:00 AM; weekly (week-end headaches); full moon;
                yearly, especially springtime (when the body undergoes
                a "spring cleaning")

                > At night; can get a second wind at night

Temperature   < Heat: of sun, room, bed (kicks off covers in bed at night
                or protrudes feet from under the covers for coolness);
                spring and summer; warm clothes or bathing

                > Cool air, breezes (wants windows open), cold bathing

Position   < Standing

                > Motion; activity; collapsing into a chair

Food/Drink   < Milk (lactose intolerance); alcohol

                > Cool drinks; great thirst for cold drinks: ice water, milk,
                carbonated beverages

                Sulphur likes most foods: sweets, salt, spices, fats (butter),
                ethnic foods, but he might dislike some specific food, such
                as cooked broccoli, brussels sprouts, spinach, liver, or
                eggs

Other   < Bathing

GUIDING MENTAL SYMPTOMS

An individual of scholarly or philosophical bent, capable of high
  achievement and strong ideas that forge the destinies of others

Strong opinions that he does not scruple to express

Entrepreneurial mentality in finance, business, etc.

Especially productive when working in an atmosphere of commotion
  (much of which he generates himself)

Can be critical of others—seldom of himself

Boastful; seeks personal recognition

The remedy picture also includes laziness and aversion to work

Egotism and selfishness; or, conversely, exceptional generosity

Quick to anger, quick to subside; erupts easily, but forgives and forgets
  easily

Generally not of a fearful disposition, but might be afraid of heights,
  or fears for the safety of loved ones (imagines disasters)

Pulsatilla

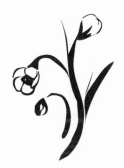

The remedy *Pulsatilla* is made from the meadow anemone, *Pulsatilla nigricans,* a plant of the Ranunculus family that grows in the plains and pasturelands of Central and Northern Europe and is commonly known as the "wind flower." It is small and delicate, with a flexible stem that bends one way or another, according to the direction of the prevailing wind.

The *Pulsatilla* personality—found predominantly in women and children—reflects this image. The initial impression is an engaging one; the woman is mild-tempered, agreeable, easy to get along with, and her sweet disposition is observed in her pretty smile, gestures, and manner or in her soft and pleasing voice. In many cases there is a corresponding sweetness of heart: delicacy of feeling, consideration of others, and a gentleness that restrains her from making any comment likely to wound another's sensibilities. By nature she is affectionate, with a strong need to be loved. To secure this love she will demonstrate strong peacemaking instincts. No one senses better than she the importance of cooperative behavior in any family or group situation, and she will do everything in her power to avoid any type of unpleasantness and maintain harmony.

The type's sweetness is also exhibited in the desire and capacity to make life pleasant for her loved ones. A *Pulsatilla* wife of an ex-

cessively demanding husband will answer her gruff mate in a soothing manner: "Of course, my love," or "You're so right, darling," "Just
as you say, my dear." The more surly his behavior, the more docile
and considerate she herself becomes, as if to compensate for his
unpleasantness. Only she could tolerate such a mate over the years
and still preserve a peaceful marriage. (At times, to be sure, the husband is the sweet *Pulsatilla* counterpart to a difficult wife.) In fact,
the sweet, conciliatory *Pulsatilla* woman has become something of a
literary stereotype; nineteenth century English literature abounds in
portraits of these soft, gentle, submissive, pretty heroines of uncertain fate (one has only to recall Dickens' gallery of *Pulsatilla* stereo-
types).

Another attractive characteristic is *Pulsatilla*'s absence of arrogance or self-righteousness. Because she is sensitive, she understands the actions of others, however different they may be from her
own. To understand is to forgive, and *Pulsatilla*, instinctively sensing
why people think and feel as they do, forgives more quickly than
she condemns. Furthermore, she is seldom overtly aggressive or imposing of her views. Her response to opposition is tears and touchiness rather than belligerence.

Pulsatilla's sweetness and desire to please do not exclude an
underlying ability to look after her own interests. Early in life she intuits that sugar catches more flies than vinegar. She likes being ca-
ressed, fussed over, and cared for. To be sure, she does not take
these signs of attention for granted but is grateful for them—graciously thanking those who help her, while offering her own affection in return as good and legal tender. For this reason, others do
not object to helping her. Often, they are even unaware of the demands she places on them (although an apparent tyrant of a husband might lament, "I don't know how it happens. My wife is com-
pliancy itself; she never insists and never argues—but somehow she
always manages to get her own way"). Consequently, the woman
can float through life as a petted, pampered child.

Despite sweet looks and manner, then, *Pulsatilla* is not all sugar.
Beneath the surface mildness lies the resilience of the meadow

anemone, with its roots planted firmly in the soil. In fact, the type calls to mind the fable of the oak and the reed, in which the two are debating which is the stronger, when a powerful squall smites the mighty oak to the ground, while the humbly bending reed remains unscathed. Prouder and more assertive natures may break sooner than the supple, yielding *Pulsatilla*. The traditional image of the aristocratic woman of the antebellum South illustrates this particular characteristic: the soft-spoken mistress of a plantation, all sweetness on the outside but pliable steel within. Gentle, yielding Melanie Wilkes in *Gone With the Wind,* with her loving nature and fine-spun courage, is a splendid literary example of *Pulsatilla's* combination of sweetness and strength.

Like the flower swaying in the wind, *Pulsatilla* is subject to changeable moods. Aptly called the "weathercock" among remedies, she can be passive one moment, lively the next; happy one hour, miserable the next. The variable energy and moods are paralleled on the physical plane by the types' pains, which wander from one part of the body to another or shift rapidly from joint to joint—with no two attacks alike. Likewise, many symptoms come on and disappear suddenly, as if brought on by a gust of wind. *Pulsatilla* has also been described as "mentally an April day," because of her lability— laughing one moment, crying the next; or, just as the sun shines through an April shower, indulging in both simultaneously. The phrase also suggests that, like the April rain that clears the air and leaves the countryside sunnier and brighter, to this type weeping is a gentle catharsis that leaves her brighter and happier afterward.

Whether consciously or unconsciously, *Pulsatilla* effectively uses her tears to disarm. In a quarrel she will burst into tears and shoulder the blame: "Yes, it's all my fault. I know I'm in the wrong, as always. I can't do anything right—Oh, I'm hopeless!" All this leaves her adversary with little choice but to wait for her to wipe her tears and to shoulder some of the blame, reassuring her that it is not all her fault.

Just as the meadow anemone is swayed by every passing

breeze, so *Pulsatilla,* responding to the passing moment and changing social environment, blows one way and another, revealing a habitual inability to make up her mind on matters both large and small. Chronically uncertain of what she wants and hesitating about what to do, even when she does decide, she may have trouble abiding by her decision. She is fatigued and unnerved by the alternatives that daily life presents.

When she shops, her equivocation becomes apparent. She will handle twenty apparently identical peaches, turning each one over in her hand, before picking four. Or, after spending an inordinate amount of time weighing the merits of different styles of wine glasses, she will ask the salesperson, "Which ones should I buy—the short sturdy ones or the taller fluted ones?" The experienced salesperson, accustomed to *Pulsatilla* shoppers, will confidently pick one style and proffer a convincing reason for it. Sometimes she will take the advice, sometimes she will do the opposite; but at least, stimulated by the voice of authority, she makes a choice. For a long time afterward, however, she might question the wisdom of her decision. Something in her nature resists that final commitment to purchase. The same happens in a restaurant, where she must choose from a list of tempting dishes. Menus bring out the worst in her, as she not only takes a long time deciding, but, having decided, invariably changes her mind several times. It is often best for someone else to order for her; the relief will be general. Or a *Pulsatilla* college student may be unable to decide on a major and will make up her mind only at the last minute, depending on which professor she likes most at the moment. Sometimes *Pulsatilla* will continue her vacillation between two men long after marriage. Even the woman who has chosen correctly may wonder about her selection ten or fifteen years later. She equivocates less out of regret (*Pulsatilla* does not regret) than from a capacity still to respond to the other emotionally. Occasionally her old vacillation surfaces in a strong internal cry of "Why couldn't I have had *both*!"

Pulsatilla's irresolution, in fact, is sometimes reminiscent of Buridan's hypothetical ass in medieval philosophy. Finding himself equidistant from two sheaves of hay of equal size, the animal remains rooted to the spot from an inability to decide which one to approach—and ultimately dies (poor thing!) of starvation. Similarly, this irresolute type finds no reason to choose one ice cream flavor, one college, one suitor over another. She sees virtues in all of them. But fortunately, she does not starve; the human *Pulsatilla* can and does voice her dilemma in a way that a mute beast could not, and someone invariably turns up to help her.

One variant of the indecisive type is worth mentioning: the individual who is forever equivocating and asking for guidance but who, in fact, is seldom influenced by the advice so assiduously sought. Advising a *Pulsatilla* can be likened to prodding an amoeba. It appears to yield but then lapses again into its original fluctuating amorphousness.

Altogether, with her docile, tractable nature and chronic indecisiveness, *Pulsatilla* gives the impression of responding to the will of others rather than controlling her own destiny. Indeed, she may go happily through life relying on another's judgment to resolve her equivocations. She is assisted in this by her innate trust in people— by her ever-willingness to give others the benefit of the doubt until they have proved themselves unworthy of trust. Here again, Melanie Wilkes, in her refusal to acknowledge (or her inability even to conceive of) any character flaws or stain of dishonor in those she loves, exemplifies this trait.

A corollary of *Pulsatilla*'s indecisiveness is her pleasing adaptability. With little heaviness or pedantry in her nature and a high degree of tolerance, she easily adapts to another's preferences or lifestyle. Intellectual and emotional flexibility are reflected in her range of tastes. She is a great appreciator of various art forms, ranging from the classical composers and painters to pottery, ethnic handcrafts, and beadwork. Receptive to the merits of all, she responds to each in the same open-minded way. When asked to name her favorite art form, she might reply, "I like them all," and even be astonished by the question. How can one art form be preferred over another? If

asked whether she prefers classical or romantic music, she will give
the same somewhat perplexed answer: "Why, I like them both!" This
is quite different from intellectually critical individuals who have
strong likes and dislikes when an art form either coincides with their
particular preferences or does not ("I like romantic poetry, but hate
modern" or "I love jazz, but hate country music"). Adapting to the
mood of another, *Pulsatilla* easily relates to any artist's vision.

Furthermore, by not making hard and fast judgments, *Pulsatilla*
remains flexible in her relations with others. In difficult or deteriorating relationships, when unable to decide what to do, she waits
and lets things slide, trusting that they will straighten out. Often they
do, thus vindicating her passive approach. In this way she may fare
better than those who quarrel in haste and break in heat, then re-
pent at leisure. The same is true of other stressful situations in life.
Her adaptability enables her to drift with the tide and adapt to cross-
currents—instead of fighting them, as more assertive natures are apt
to do.

This trait introduces another prominent *Pulsatilla* characteristic—companionability. Just as the meadow anemone grows in clus-
ters, so the human *Pulsatilla* enjoys having people around her. She
loves companionship of all kinds: the young and the old, the boring and the amusing, the intense and the serene. Not only is she
friendly, affectionate, and inherently well-disposed toward others,
but also, by virtue of being one of the least critical constitutional
types, she harbors an openness toward her fellow humans that allows her easily to empathize with them, to enter into all details of
their lives and be sincerely interested in hearing about their children,
homes, health, and hobbies. She possesses a naturally civilized manner, with an ability to detect nuances of feeling and to sense the
niceties of thought without needing to have them elucidated. Additionally, she displays an instinctive sense for when to talk and when
to listen, so that after the initial shyness she relates naturally and
effortlessly; and in her accepting presence, others feel thoroughly
comfortable.

Pulsatilla's talent for relating to others is undeniably a virtue
and a strength. But her yielding and obliging disposition has a pragmatic aspect as well. She takes pains to cultivate an extensive network of friends who will always be at hand, ready to respond, when
she sends out the call. Discord is to be avoided, both because she
relies on others' moods to be happy herself and because it would
cut her off from some part of her supportive network. Consequently,
the other side of the coin of *Pulsatilla*'s companionability is dependence. She is not (as noted earlier) intrinsically fragile or weak, but
just as ivy seeks out a supporting wall or tree, so *Pulsatilla* seeks
someone on whom to lean. In her very voice there is an easily recognized imploring or beseeching "Will you help me? *Please,* tell me
what to do!" tone. Indeed, the type's particular appealing or delicate
quality stems in part from this perceptible, almost tangible, need for
support.

Pulsatilla is attractive to men, possessing as she does that
sweetness that is so highly valued by them as the evidence of female
worth and a manner that flatters the male ego. She is nonthreatening
and, in her obvious search for a supportive shoulder, makes a man
feel strong, useful, indispensable—and, consequently, good about
himself. Men instinctively want to reach out, hold, and protect her.
Sometimes even several men may be willing to take on the responsibility of surrounding her throughout life with a protective hedge.
Wind flower that she is, she blows this way and that, not knowing
whom to choose and wishing she could marry more than one. But
once she has found stability in family life, she is entirely fulfilled and
remains a faithful, affectionate wife and satisfied mother. Many a
happy marriage has resulted because the spouse is largely *Pulsatilla*
in character.

Such dependence on the opposite sex is no female monopoly:
the man who requires the support of one, and sometimes two,
strong women to get through life is often a *Pulsatilla*. Yet women do
not object to such dependence. Not only does the essentially sweet
nature of the son, brother, husband, or lover bring out all their protective and maternal instincts, but also the *Pulsatilla* man does give

something in return for the support he seeks. Like the woman, he gives affection and offers the opportunity for a warm, pleasant, close relationship.

There was much of this remedy, for example, in composer Felix Mendelssohn. Born to an easy, protected, and privileged life, and the pet of his affectionate family, he was famous for his sweet disposition (reflected in the intensely lyrical quality of his music) that enabled him to get along exceptionally well with family, friends, and even fellow musicians. Memoirs of his contemporaries attest to his invariable gentleness and absence of egotism—astounding in a composer of his magnitude. Moreover, *three* good women cared for him throughout his life: mother, sister, and later, his wife. He was so attached to all of them that his mother's death brought on an illness that severely weakened him, and the news of his sister's death shortly afterward, when he was only thirty-eight, caused a relapse and a stroke from which his delicate constitution never recovered.

Thus, *Pulsatilla* is happy living in a situation in which she can share her life and responsibilities with others. Because she is compliant, she abides by the rules and is a reliable contributing member of her chosen circle. Because she instinctively recognizes the need for tolerance and give-and-take in a family or group, she readily accedes to the will of others and works harmoniously with them.

Not only is *Pulsatilla* receptive to influence and guidance, she also requires someone to listen to her woes in troubled times and a friendly shoulder to cry on. The very act of confiding in another, of pouring out her problems in long heart-to-heart talks with half a dozen people from her supportive network, restores her emotional equilibrium. Trusting, dependent, confiding, she truly believes that others can offer solace and assist her—so of course they do.

However, in her dependence, *Pulsatilla* may place severe demands on the time, solicitude, and emotional reserves of those willing to help her. In family or amorous relationships and even friendships, she seeks ever more support, ever more reassurance of being loved, until at length, others feel they are captives. At first they want to reach out in compassion, with a "Poor thing, let me help you" impulse—which she allows; but with time, the clinging can become burdensome. In her tender affection she entwines others in soft tendrils, but the clutching tendrils are chains nonetheless. Those wishing to withdraw their support are beset by feelings of guilt. They fear that the ivy can no longer be separated from the supporting wall without being destroyed

Pulsatilla is also prone to self-pity. Here again, the very inflection of her voice, the sweet and slightly plaintive "You're hurting my feelings—don't you know how sensitive I am?" announces this trait. Sensitive plant that she is, she is easily wounded, and her self-pity may lead her to feel offended in a situation in which another would laugh. The following example is indicative. A man was describing his wife's tendency to offer a bewildering variety of choices to guests at dinner parties: "Would you like your vegetables now or later? And what about salad—on a separate plate from the meat or the same? Should I put gravy on your potatoes, or do you want to take some yourself?" The incident was recounted humorously and not unkindly, but the wife was hurt and remonstrated plaintively, "I was only trying to make everyone happy, to give them just what they wanted. You know how sensitive I am about people—"

"But people don't *want* so many choices," the husband interrupted. "They prefer to be served food on their plates and not to have to make endless decisions whether to have whole-wheat or white rolls, salad now or later, take regular or herbal tea. Just give them something, and most of them will be happy—or *should* be at any rate!"

"Oh," the woman mewed self-pityingly, "I guess I never will be able to get things right. But I *do* try. And if you would only help me instead of always criticizing, it would be so much easier. And if only I weren't so sensitive about everybody and everything. . . ." and she relapsed into a familiar *Pulsatilla* plaint about her sensitivity.

On a more serious level, originating as a means to gain sympathy and support, self-pity can imperceptibly erode the morale and prevent *Pulsatilla* from facing up maturely to life's reversals.

Pulsatilla is essentially nonintellectual. Ruled by her sensibilities and influenced by her emotions, the mentality is appreciative rather than authoritarian, and she feels more comfortable dealing with the particulars of everyday life and human relations rather than with intellectual theories and abstractions. In conversation she seeks above all to establish a pleasant friendly rapport; the larger concepts or factual information are of secondary concern. Following Jung's classification of the human personality into four types—the sensory, intellectual, emotional, and intuitive—*Pulsatilla* falls squarely into the emotional category. Thus, she systematically brings generalities down to the personal level and interprets abstractions in the light of her own feelings, preferences, or experience. For instance, if someone mentions the increased violence in the world, she will remark that her Jenny was being increasingly picked on by playmates in the park. Or, in a general discussion of the relative merits of boarding versus day school, she will comment, "I would never send *my* son to boarding school. I feel we have too much to offer him here at home."

One typically *Pulsatilla* girl—pretty, sweet-mannered, gentle-voiced—during a college course discussion of Ophelia's character in Shakespeare's *Hamlet,* raised her hand and volunteered, "I can *really* relate to Ophelia."

"Yes," the instructor inquired encouragingly, eager to draw out the hitherto silent, shy girl's ideas, "in what way?"

"Well, my last boyfriend was *exactly* like Hamlet! Let me tell you how he . . ." She then went on to describe their relationship in such intimate terms that the instructor wished he had not asked.

One final observation: whatever her innate abilities (and they can be considerable), *Pulsatilla* may lack confidence in her own intellectual capacities. Blossoming as she does only under others' continuous assurances and encouragement, forever fluctuating in her feelings, she needs others' convictions to give shape and form to her ideas.

A fine literary example of the highly personal and nonintellectual nature of *Pulsatilla* is Clarissa Dalloway in Virginia Woolf's novel *Mrs. Dalloway*. The whole flow of associations in this homogeneous work (where the reader lives through the sights and sounds of a day in London) carries a *Pulsatilla* hue. First of all, Mrs. Dalloway needs to be around people on whose good opinion she depends and on whose companionship she thrives. Acutely sensitive to what others are thinking or feeling, she responds with sympathy and kindness to everyone—her family, acquaintances, servants, even a sales girl in a flower shop—wanting them all to be happy so that she can be happy herself. By the same token, she rejects any intrusive misery (as in the person of her daughter's resentful and pathetically unattractive tutor) that threatens her comfortable, civilized existence, especially her carefully cultivated serenity. Moreover, *Pulsatilla*'s nonintellectual response to the world is reflected in Mrs. Dalloway's inability to recall whether her husband was on a committee to help the Albanians or the Armenians (they were all the same to her)—reminiscent of Disraeli's *Pulsatilla* wife, who claimed she could never remember who came first, the Greeks or the Romans. In true *Pulsatilla* fashion, Clarissa Dalloway appreciates the passionate impulses, mercurial nature, and ironic mind of her rejected suitor, Peter Walsh, no less than the emotional delicacy, integrity, and sense of service of her reserved husband. Thus, she remains reliant on the affection and approval of both. Further, in her finely fluctuating moods, Mrs. Dalloway responds with exquisite sensitivity to all external impressions: the sky, the flowers, the sound of the clock striking the hour, the sight of a billowing curtain—as she weaves in and out of the minds and feelings of the small group of characters around whom the novel revolves.

All in all, *Pulsatilla* has a pleasing, prepossessing nature—mild, malleable, kindly disposed and nonaggressive, with a sincere wish to accommodate, true consideration of others' feelings, and a charitable rather than a censorious attitude toward humanity. There is strength in her sociable and sensitive (even if at times self-pitying) disposition, in her yielding and adaptable nature. After all, it was the massive oak that was laid low by the North Wind, not the fragile yet resilient reed. And if one bears in mind the characteristics just discussed—sweetness, flexibility, companionability, dependence, and a gentle emotionalism—one should seldom fail to recognize, especially in women, the picture of the delicate and beautiful meadow anemone.

Pulsatilla

PRINCIPAL REGIONS AFFECTED

Head	Headache from overwork; wandering stitches in the head, neuralgic pains; pains extend to face and teeth; eyes agglutinated; **conjunctivitis;** blepharitis; **tears flow easily** (from wind, cold); **earaches;** ears feel stuffed; diminished hearing acuity; discharges
Digestion	Heaviness, discomfort, or pain (one hour after eating); loose stool; **no two stools alike**
Male	**Swelling and inflammation of the organs; enlarged prostate**
Female	**Cystitis:** difficulties urinating; interrupted urine stream; urine passes only in drops; with burning; stress incontinence; creamy, acrid vaginal discharges; **premenstrual symptoms;** painful menses, with headache, back pains; menstrual flow clotted, changeable, intermittent; diarrhea before, during, or after; menses suppressed, delayed, or tardy at puberty; menopausal hot flashes, palpitations, night sweats; **complaints of pregnancy, childbirth, and lactation:** morning sickness; breech position; false, delayed, or weak labor; retained placenta; milk scanty or too profuse; difficulties weaning
Extremities	Swollen and painful joints (especially lower limbs); **varicose veins**

GENERALITIES

Symptoms forever changing: shifting from one side to another or wandering from place to place

Variable temperature; flushes up and gets heated easily; also easily chilled

Pulsating, throbbing, or jerking nature of pains and symptoms

Thick, bland, yellow or greenish-yellow discharges (from eyes or nose; of expectoration and leukorrhea)

Sound sleep in the morning, hard to waken; **wakens tired and unrefreshed;** numbness of parts lain on during sleep

Difficulty falling asleep from restlessness or some persistent thought running through the mind

Vivid dreams of day's difficulties, or frightening ones (i.e., being pursued by a black animal); but also agreeable dreams

When first impairment of health is referred to age of puberty

Continued.

Pulsatilla—cont'd

MODALITIES (< worse; > better)

Time	< Morning, upon awakening; evening; **alternate days**
Temperature	< **Heat of sun**; stuffy rooms, warm bed and clothes (even if chilly)
	> **Cool breezes**, cold bathing and applications of cold; open air
Position	< Sitting or standing still; beginning motion; **lying on left or painful side**
	> **Gentle and continued motion (walking)**; lying with head high, arms thrown above the head
Food/Drink	< **Rich and fatty food; pork; eating late at night**
	> Cool drinks
	Desire for desserts, pastry, butter (even if it disagrees)
	Generally **thirstless**
Other	> **Pouring out her troubles; after a good cry; sympathy and consolation**

GUIDING MENTAL SYMPTOMS

Sweet disposition, affectionate, yielding, sensitive to others' feelings

Shyness, timidity

Docile and dependent; wants to be influenced: relies on others

Highly emotional; **changeable moods; emotionally a "weathercock";** indecisiveness

Tearful, self-pitying, whiny state alternates with cheerfulness

Fears of being alone in the evening; of the dark; of ghosts; **making decisions, independence;** of opposite sex or of people in general (shyness); of **being emotionally hurt**

Arsenicum album

> Anything worth doing is worth overdoing.
>
> —Anonymous

The above epigraph points straight to the heart of *Arsenicum album* and is a continuing theme in the picture of this strong, projecting, and, for the most part, driven personality.

What is the source of *Arsenicum*'s drive? For what is he striving? The answer is: *perfection.* He is the perfectionist par excellence; he himself admits it. But perfection is seldom achieved in this world, even by *Arsenicum* himself, hence his unceasing, unrelenting drive.

The aspiration to perfection begins early in life and can already be perceived in the child, who is unusually persevering and conscientious. This picture is continued in the pale, exhausted model student who, not satisfied with simply receiving good grades through moderate effort, must obtain the best grades through superior effort. One college student explained that he had to *over*prepare for every examination, because if he did not know the answer to even one question in ten, his mental faculties were so paralyzed that he could not concentrate on the other nine. Besides, however serious the physical consequences of such overexertion, they were still preferable to the anxiety of feeling not fully prepared.

The same striving for perfection is found in the adult, who labors indefatigably to master a new discipline or works compulsively on a project he has set his mind to—adding to it, tearing it apart, then reconstructing it, never completely satisfied with what he has done. He sleeps poorly as a consequence, and other aspects of his life must give way to the project that currently engrosses him, but still he is unable to slow down or go on to the next thing, because he cannot live with an unfinished product or an unmastered skill.

And there is more to the picture: although in seeking perfection *Arsenicum* may drive himself to exhaustion, hard work gives him immense satisfaction. After all, he is not one to put himself out unless he so chooses, knowing full well how to take care of his own comfort and interests ("I'm one helluva hard worker," he says cheerfully of himself). The more responsibility piled on him, the happier he is—in this way exemplifying the popular wisdom in the business world that a job needing to be done quickly and well should be given to the busiest person in the office (that is, to an *Arsenicum*). Thus, the overzealous, overconscientious, unrelenting businessman, lawyer, doctor, or broker who works long hours without let-up and is then unable to unwind—who accomplishes as much in one day as any two other people, yet still reproaches himself for not accomplishing enough—is often an *Arsenicum*. Other constitutional types may possess a similar capacity for and enjoyment of work, but it is *Arsenicum*'s driven, compulsive manner that makes him unique.

Although his colossal inner drive creates the semblance of strength, he is sustained more by nervous energy than by true endurance. "I often feel as if I am running full speed on 'below empty,'" was one individual's way of phrasing it, as he oscillated between excessive application and total exhaustion. Yet, barely recovered from a collapse, he starts up again on all cylinders. For the truth of the matter is that the ultra-ambitious and overachieving *Arsenicum* is not content unless he is pushing himself to the limits of his strength.

He may actually suffer from headaches on weekends when unable to go to the office to work. Some will fall ill during vacations or become restless and irascible while relaxing at the seashore; they cannot wait to get back to the daily grind. When under stress, at a low point in life, or in a state of despair, *Arsenicum*'s most reliable and effective therapy—his panacea—is to immerse himself in work. For certain individuals work may even take the place of an emotional life. They find in it the pleasure and meaning that other constitutional types find only in human relations.

Arsenicum's driven quality may prevent him from resting on his laurels and enjoying his own achievements. Highly self-critical and with his eye always fixed on some distant peak, a triumph or a success is merely one more step in an endless progression of (largely self-imposed) compulsory achievements. No accomplishment can calm his drive, because it comes from within and is not satisfied by the world's acclaim. To be sure, he seeks acknowledgment as much as another and will not turn it down when it is deserved, but this is neither his primary motive nor his principal source of satisfaction. Always looking toward the next goal, he presses ever forward.

This driven perfectionist can also be seen in family situations, especially in the female *Arsenicum*. At best she is the "supermom" who balances the needs of husband, children, career, and household without impairing the interests of any. In her well-regulated life she finds time to do everything (including playing an active role on the school board or the Neighborhood Watch committee), and every minute of her day is accounted for. Although this may require tight deadlines and rigid adherence to plans drawn up and enforced by her restless energy, she uses the time efficiently and everything is done well, without missing a beat. She is a fair-minded disciplinarian and intelligently supportive parent, with happy, creative, and well-balanced children.

At times, however, the *"Arsenicum* mother" caricatures the type. Eager to promote her children's welfare, she assails doctors, teachers, friends, and relatives with importunate demands. Her relentless drive for perfection may lead her to transfer her child from one school to another in midterm, yank him out of an extracurricular activity in which he is perfectly content and enroll him in another, or constantly switch tutors, doctors, and babysitters, while frankly indicating to each his deficiencies and the reasons for the change. Bulldozing all obstacles before her, she clears the ground for her children to follow—and woe betide anyone who stands in her path!

Sometimes this pushy mother's overly high expectations can operate to the detriment of the children or lead to a poor relationship with them. This is exhibited in the constantly scolding mother who is impatient with her children's weaknesses, quick to badger them or show her disappointment, and when discontent with their performance, berates them in that peculiarly *Arsenicum* no-let-up "dentist drill" style. A grown child's observation about such a critical parent is, "I now realize that *nothing* I could have ever done—or been—would have satisfied her [or him]."

Some *Arsenicum* individuals exhibit the same relentless perfectionism toward their health. In striving for absolute good health, they spare no effort (insisting that all around them cooperate in their exertions), cultivating it with such eagerness and ardor as leaves others nonplussed. Not being in perfect health seems to *Arsenicum* incomprehensible, illogical, and totally unjust.

This trait of carrying a good thing to excess in matters of health is often directed at various kinds of diets. The *Arsenicum* individual almost invariably holds strong opinions about the correct kinds and quantity of food that is essential for maintaining optimum health. He will religiously follow the most Spartan regimen and delights in nutritional fads. He may undergo rigorous fasts and restrictive diets over an extended period, oblivious to the dangers of depriving himself of essential nutrients. This is the person who indeed does not live by bread alone, but by his interminable theories on nutrition.

Terribly ambitious as *Arsenicum* is to achieve perfection and to be "the best," he can display a strong competitiveness. Whether subtly or in an assertive way, he must constantly prove himself better than others. The student obsessed with grades and who talks about them endlessly is often *Arsenicum*—as is the individual who builds himself up by criticizing others. There is room at the top for only one person—himself—and he brooks no competition there. In any situation, exchange of ideas, or relationship, he cannot resist being one jump ahead of others. Within the family, a proud father will say of his son's good report card, "All A minuses, that's wonderful! But when I was your age, I used to bring home all A's!" The parent who tires others with endless glowing accounts of his children's varied talents, virtues, and accomplishments is often exhibiting *Arsenicum*'s innate competitiveness. Everything "belonging" to him or her—children, spouse, job, house, garden—must be superlative, and better than anyone else's. Even his illnesses must be more interesting or serious than others'.

On the other hand, some ambitious *Arsenicums* will manifest a disarming lack of competitiveness. They want only to excel themselves and have no objection if others excel also. A child will run home from school very excited that twelve members of his class (including himself) got an A on a math test. Or a ballet teacher who is driving her aspiring daughter to high achievement will drive her other students equally; she wants them all to become great ballerinas. This individual will honestly enjoy and generously applaud a performance or accomplishment superior to his own. He is enthralled by perfection—however and in whomever it may be manifested.

To achieve (and especially maintain) perfection, an individual must have full control over his environment as well as over himself. Whether obvious about it or inconspicuous, *Arsenicum* is a controlling personality who takes the lead in personal relations, determining their scope and tone, balancing the give and take, and leaving others no choice but to comply. In virtually all circumstances, this domineering individual cannot abide others being in charge and insists on making all decisions himself. Quite unable simply to sit back and let things follow their natural course, he needs to oversee and run everything himself.

As an employer his self-drive impels him to drive others—pushing for more, bigger, better. Impatient at delays, quick to feel frustration, he often wants to dance faster than the music—that is, accelerate the course of events and others' responses to them. He can be overanxious, overwatchful, and incapable of delegating responsibility. He checks and rechecks what others have done, tells them exactly how they should do something, or, if they have done it, how they should have done it differently. Even in the home, whether in preparing a meal or putting up the storm windows, others are merely allowed (or expected) to assist by following his directions. His spouse laments that she feels as if she were an indentured servant who must, by obedience and submission in work, justify her right to live in her own home. Likewise, the *Arsenicum* housewife hangs around the kitchen giving ceaseless instructions to her dutiful husband or child or any person trying to be helpful. She may disapprove of the way the dishes are stacked in the dishwasher and must immediately rearrange them "better." She is notorious for frantically tidying up her house the day before the cleaning woman arrives. Instead of relaxing on this one day, she drives herself into a harassed and irritable frenzy. She offers many justifications for this behavior, but the ultimate reason is her inability to relinquish control. In extreme cases she will follow the unfortunate cleaning woman around, supervising her every step.

In general, *Arsenicum* takes pride in his ability to grapple with the varied problems of everyday life and in giving good advice to others. He or she loves putting people's houses in order—either literally (these people make the best housekeepers) or figuratively. The superefficient junior colleague or employee who always knows better than his superiors and insists on running the show his own way is *Arsenicum*—as is the secretary who rearranges her employer's files more efficiently or the editor who is superb at whipping into shape an article, a short story, or novel written by someone else.

By the same token, his love of control, combined with a tendency to be ultracritical of others' performance, makes this type the best of teachers—since teaching furnishes him with an admirable occasion for dictating to others. Completely dedicated to his profession, never tiring of shaping and molding others, he unsparingly imparts his sound knowledge and critical talents to his students. In private instruction (such as language and music lessons), *Arsenicum* can be the sternest of taskmasters: supportive of good work, but impatient with poor preparation and chary with compliments. "It's coming along," he will comment on a piece of music well performed; or, as the supreme accolade, "It plays well!" He does not aim to discourage, and secretly he is proud of the student who reflects his own good teaching, but, always looking ahead, he wants to elevate him to an even higher level of achievement. Those two incomparable teachers, Leopold (father of Mozart) and Annie Sullivan (the guide of Helen Keller), who steered (not to say drove) their charges to genius, were undoubtedly *Arsenicums*. At times, then, this individual seeks to control not only the present but also the future. The ambitious mother in the well-known joke, who introduces her three sons, aged seven, five, and three, "The oldest is the lawyer, the middle one the doctor, and the youngest is the financier!" is *Arsenicum*.

To feel confident about dictating to others entails a certain amount of pride—a characteristic with which *Arsenicum* is generously endowed. "I'm always right" or "I usually know what's going on before anyone else," are typical thoughts, if not actually expressed phrases. And he often is—and does. Also, even if an elitist in his opinions, tastes, and judgments, he is more than willing to take on the responsibilities that accompany the assumption of superiority; and generally his elitism judges people less on birth, wealth, or privilege than on performance. He expects others to perform well and is consequently intolerant of mediocrity or mistakes. He forgets that, unlike himself, others may not choose to excel in some chosen field; and above all, that he himself is not exempt from his share of misjudgments. For example, Emma Woodhouse, the heroine of Jane Austen's *Emma*, thinks her judgment infallible and enjoys running other people's lives, even to the point of matchmaking. She is undoubtedly of superior intelligence, with a generous and high-minded character, yet her intellectual pride and her assumption of superiority lead her to misguided assessments of those around her and ultimately into error.

Finally, the *Arsenicum* need for control emerges full force in the health-conscious individual who conducts his life along some strictly

regulated routine, adjusted precisely to suit his physical and emotional needs. The authoritarian *Arsenicum* likes regulation, authority,
and discipline so much that if others do not impose it on him, he
will impose it on himself. He may push himself mercilessly to run
several miles each day, even in the most inclement weather, or in
other ways to stay physically fit. And his dietary precautions are
proverbial. One memorable individual would bring not only his own
tea when visiting, but even his own teapot—made from a special
clay that, he claimed, was imperative for his well-being. Moreover,
this is the patient who feels compelled to tell his various physicians
(he usually has a legion of them caring for him) what each one has
said, or not said, about his complaint—pointing out what they had
done wrong and advising the current doctor what he thinks is the
correct procedure. *Arsenicum,* in short, must be on top of every situation: directing it, overseeing it, and commanding others in order to
achieve a perfect end result.

Because no person can exert complete control over his life and
environment, *Arsenicum* succumbs to various fears. Among the
most fearful of personality types, he is beset with anxieties reasonable and unreasonable, tangible and intangible, major and minor,
present and future, visible and hidden. Even when he claims to be
(and is) depressed, he projects less an aura of sadness and dejection
than of anxiety and frustration. His anxiety may be exhibited in
some specific worry, or in a general mental restlessness and antici-
pation of troubles—or it manifests as perfectionism and authoritari-
anism and in a tendency to immoderation or extremism.

For instance, in his desire for order, discipline, and superior performance, *Arsenicum* becomes terribly upset when the unexpected
occurs and he must adjust to unforeseen circumstances. Likewise,
his anxieties surface when others fail to comply with his well-
thought-through plans. (Alas, perfection has once more eluded him!)
Here too, when complaining that nothing is being done right, he
does not take into account that others might not want to operate
with his fanatical precision; nor do they derive his level of enjoy-

ment from consummating intricate schemes through superior efficiency, organization, and split-second timing. Predictably, one of his
anxieties and concerns is punctuality. Haunted by fears of being late,
he takes no chances. He starts out for his destination in plenty of
time, allowing for delays on the road, and often arrives far too early
for appointments ("I am pathologically prompt," he readily admits).
And, of course, he begins packing for a short journey hours in advance.

One of *Arsenicum*'s most common anxieties is safety. This is
quite a prominent feature. A woman may be perpetually worried
that something will happen to her husband or children and grows
frantic if one of them stays out fifteen minutes longer than expected.
She wears herself out by imagining some dreadful occurrence, en-
acting the whole scene in her mind, down to the last detail. She will
drive her preteen child five blocks to school when all the other children walk or bicycle, since this is preferable to sitting at home
worrying whether he got there safely. Even public transportation for
after-school activities is out of the question. She cannot sleep at
night until her teenage children are home from a party and lies
awake thinking of all the terrible possibilities. The *Arsenicum* man is
equally full of fears: every time he steps in the car, he thinks of accidents and fatalities. Even on a short trip, he fears that he may never
see his wife and children again.

Money is another source of concern to *Arsenicum*. Whether or
not he has it, he thinks and talks about it a great deal, frequently
lamenting his poverty or the high cost of living. He can be tight with
a dollar—easily resisting impulses to lend it, disliking to spend it
even when he has it, and claiming not to be able to afford some perfectly affordable article or necessary expense. Always a conscientious worker, he develops his talents unsparingly so as to become
indispensable at his job. He might even devote evenings, weekends,
and vacations to acquiring a second skill as a second source of in-
come, for fear of future financial need. He is no mere jack-of-all-
trades, as *Sulphur* frequently is, but rather is the master of several,
and likes to keep at least two strings to his bow at all times.

But by far the most striking of *Arsenicum*'s anxieties is health. Aside from his perfectionist's frustration at the malfunctioning of any part of his anatomy, he is terrified by the prospect of losing control over his own body. He becomes fearful of setbacks, relapses, or delays in the process of cure and fights illness with such vehemence as serves only to exacerbate his condition and hinder cure. Even in minor ailments he grows frantic at the very thought of insubordination by some organ, lamenting, "I'm doing everything I should—eating right, exercising every day, taking good care of myself—but still I don't feel well. What *am* I doing wrong?" Conversely, the healthy *Arsenicum* talks with pride of being always "in control" of his body.

His physical well-being, or lack of same, is thus a source of endless and all-absorbing interest. He regards his illness with disproportionate dread (for instance, a puffiness under the eyes upon awakening in the morning is magnified beyond its real importance), panics at symptoms that others would ignore, and naturally, imagines he has every disease he reads about. In an excited voice he will tell of a recent book by some "wonderfully insightful physician, who has pointed out to me a number of important problems that I never *knew* I had until I read his book. What an incredible medical mind the man has!"

In safeguarding his health and controlling his fears, *Arsenicum* often carries regimens and precautions to amazing lengths. Allowing for no exceptions or compromises, he consumes dozens of medicinal or vitamin pills daily and avoids whole lists of benign foods as if they were pure poison. Not surprisingly, in view of the fact that the remedy is made from arsenic, *Arsenicum* displays an inordinate fear of being poisoned by bad food. He will not leave food outside the refrigerator for even a short time, convinced that it will spoil. If a piece of cheese is moldy, he throws it away instead of simply scraping off the mold. The *Arsenicum* housewife becomes suspicious of something she has just prepared, deciding that it smells funny, or tastes strange, or looks off-color. Ever on the alert for contaminated food, she threatens to throw away the entire dish, to the horror of her hungry family. The type is also excessively anxious about germs and contagion. Perceiving pollution and imminent decay on all sides, he will, through constant cleaning, scrubbing, and germicidal sprays, combat them every way he can.

For all his dread of illness, the type is fascinated by medicine (it is not by chance that *Arsenicum* is exceptionally highly represented in the medical profession) and loves doctors. Not only does he never tire of talking about his health and illnesses, he willingly undergoes innumerable medical workups and laboratory tests—many of which are of questionable necessity. He travels miles from one physician to another, trying therapy after therapy, as he seeks both confirmation of the seriousness of his complaint and reassurance of its curability. He likes nothing better than to visit a holistic health clinic, where he can with justification patronize six practitioners (a nutritionist, chiropractor, massage therapist, homoeopath, psychotherapist, and an acupuncturist) and undergo six types of treatments almost simultaneously. He may be right to take responsibility for his well-being, but sometimes the effort is disproportionate. Instead of pursuing his goal of good health merely sufficiently to live a productive life, he allows it to become virtually an obsession and his *raison d'être.*

To do the type justice, however, there often is a legitimate basis for his anxiety with regard to health. *Arsenicum* can be likened to the *E*-string on the violin—the thinnest, tautest, and most delicately tuned of all the strings, which is not only the source of the most sensitive vibrations but also the first to go out of tune. Either it snaps from the least excess of tension or, if strung a fraction of a millimeter too loose, it plays flat. In just the same way, *Arsenicum* must be perfectly adjusted to function well. That means the physical environment must be just right for this individual who is inherently allergy and/or asthma prone and who displays numerous sensitivities: to various foods; to dust, mold, feathers, or animal hair and dander; to odors; to sounds (the slightest of which may prevent sleep); to cold (or any temperature outside his two- to three-degree tolerance range). And building up a supportive environment does, in truth, require much care and concern on his part.

Altogether, *Arsenicum*'s anxieties have a restless, persistent quality to them. Terrier-like, he worries every issue or concern to death. If not anxious about the present, he worries about the near or distant future. He is not certain when or where the sword of Damocles will fall, but fall it must, and he is thus alert at all times. His mind may be so preoccupied with his various fears that the happy resolution of one problem merely leaves a vacuum to be filled by the next.

Returning to the theme of perfection: people are not perfect, human performance is imperfect, nature is far from perfect, scientific theories are always being reinterpreted and supplanted by newer ones, and ideas of ethics and morality or of politics and religion are continually changing—so that what is truth today may be falsehood tomorrow. Only in art, *Arsenicum* concludes, can perfection be attained—and even more important, sustained. Consequently, the type is often attracted to the creative arts and ranks high in the constitutional economy of writers, painters, sculptors, and composers. Even if belonging primarily to another constitutional type, these individuals invariably display a prominent *Arsenicum* streak as well. The remedy picture is also found in those who might be called disguised artists: seamstresses, gardeners, hairdressers, surgeons, gourmet cooks, and the like—all occupations requiring an artistic touch to mold something perfect out of the material given.

That which helps *Arsenicum* excel in the creative arts is an innate meticulousness and his infinite capacity for taking pains. He loves precision and concentration on detail—and is able to stick with the matter at hand until the desired objective is achieved, no matter how long it takes. For this reason, he is also often encountered in the constitutional composition of performing artists. Although tense and nervous throughout the performance, he is carried to the top by his ambition, willingness to train and practice long hours, and above all by his unflagging drive for perfection. This is what sustains him in the arduous—at times slavelike—labor of the performing artist; and conceivably such a career, in turn, brings out or develops the *Arsenicum* side in an individual.

It is, however, more than mere personal ambition that compels this type to put himself out to the extent he does for whatever he undertakes to accomplish. He is being driven by his sense of what is due to those out there counting on his expertise and expecting from him a high standard of performance. He *owes* it to others to live up to their expectations; the artist in him is ever seeking to enrich life not only for himself but also for others. Indeed, he owes it to the art itself—or to the science, profession, or scholarly discipline in which he is engaged (since the intellectual powers are, naturally, cultivated with the same vigor and assiduity as the artistic ones). Additionally, offer him a new challenge in his particular field, and he goes for it—with a zeal!—surmounts it, then looks around expectantly for further challenges. It is, in fact, this very quality of dedication beyond the call of duty that gives to *Arsenicum*'s work its signal power.

An applicant was one of thirty for the post of professor of music history and theory at a local university. As part of the hiring process he had to present a one-hour sample lecture to the faculty, and he resolved to analyze a movement of a Haydn sonata. He arrived with a suitcase containing (1) a tape of the work for the university audio equipment, (2) his own cassette recorder, together with a cassette, in case the university equipment was not functioning properly, (3) an outline of his lecture and a detailed syllabus of his prospective course for the entire year—in sufficient copies for everyone present, and (4) an additional tape reel, cassette, and photocopied handouts of a lecture on a Chopin prelude, in case the faculty preferred that to Haydn. He then proceeded with his lucid analysis and elegant exposition of the subject—every word weighed, every phrase balanced. This was the superorganized *Arsenicum,* prepared for every eventuality and a model of conscientious preparation. (He was the candidate chosen.)

In fiction the *Arsenicum* cast of mind is exemplified by Conan Doyle's Sherlock Holmes, the famous sleuth who has become a byword for meticulous observation, scrupulous attention to detail, and precision in analysis and deduction. Undeniably an artist in his chosen field and, true to type, standing at the top of his profession, he is also the confirmed *Arsenicum* bachelor who is devoted first and foremost to his profession—claiming that emotion will only interfere with the carefully cultivated objectivity and machinelike efficiency of his mental processes. His attitude toward Dr. Watson is also characteristic—loyal but demanding, waxing impatient at the latter's occasional slowness and incompetence ("You *see,* Watson, but you do not *observe!*" he continually rebukes his friend)—as is his self-assessment: "I cannot agree with those who rank modesty among the virtues. To the logician all things should be seen exactly as they are, and to underrate one's self is as much a departure from truth as to exaggerate one's own powers" (*The Greek Interpreter*). Then, too, in typical *Arsenicum* fashion, Holmes fluctuates between excess of nervous energy when the chase is on (during which time he can go for days without food or sleep) and collapse (into a state of bored lassitude) once the case has been solved. Even his appearance is revealing: thin, pale, ascetic-looking, with a beaked aristocratic nose in a gaunt face; long, sensitive fingers that so beautifully caress a violin; and especially those gimlet eyes, whose penetrating glance overlooks nothing.

Actually, in any sphere *Arsenicum* displays meticulousness and a sensitivity to disorder. He will fuss over the towels on the bathroom rack, hanging them straight and symmetrically. He cannot tolerate a chair that is not aligned with the table or a book that has not been reshelved in its proper place; he is upset if a picture is not hanging straight on the wall or if his shoes on the closet floor are not neatly lined up in rows according to color. He is indignant when cars are parked crookedly on the lines in parking lots ("Why can't people do it the right way? It's just as easy to park *in* the spaces") and will spend much time packing and repacking a suitcase so that everything fits together in a particular way. Although hurrying to leave for the airport, he is still atwitter about his clothes being folded neatly and socks properly paired off. In an admirable but at times excessive concern for immaculateness, the housewife constantly cleans and tidies around the house, picking up bits of thread from the carpet, wiping off fluffs of dirt from the furniture; otherwise, she cannot bear to look at it. A businessman's desk is a model of neatness and order: everything must have its designated place and be arranged in some precise manner; otherwise, he is distraught and unable to function properly. (Naturally, the gender roles can be reversed.)

Even without undue neuroses or excess, *Arsenicum* is fastidious. Both men and women are, as a rule, well dressed and meticulously groomed. The house is well appointed, the decor stylish. In fact, elegance and good taste is the hallmark of this individual; his every movement and gesture is often remarkably delicate and precise. Whether building a table or repairing a fence, cleaning the yard or painting the house, writing a report or cooking a meal, his work manifests those particular finishing touches, that final polish, that betrays the type.

Arsenicum demands much of life but can also give much to the world in return. This is the person who, holding high standards, can be counted upon to do things competently; whose intolerance of mediocrity and imperfection raises others (as well as himself) to higher levels of performance and more distinguished achievement; and who, when especially gifted, is able to bring to humanity so much beauty and joy. Moreover, not every *Arsenicum* is an anxious, domineering, excessively critical, or demanding personality. He can be the very antithesis: self-contained, pleasant to deal with, and exceptionally thoughtful of others—his high intelligence enabling him to perform socially and professionally with a happy ease.

Sometimes the tranquil disposition results from accepting some calming philosophy and reflects a deliberate subjection of his driving, controlling impulses. His behavior, after all, is largely motivated by the particular image of perfection he has adopted and that he strives to attain. At other times, however, a course of potentized arsenic is required to appease his excessive apprehensions and anxieties, to subdue any inordinate tendency to control his environment and the people around him, or to moderate his propensity (in his drive for perfection) to overdo whatever he undertakes. In either case, once *Arsenicum* has succeeded in poising himself for the accomplishments he so deeply desires—and especially once he has accepted a given balance of control and compliance in a relationship, he can be recognized in the gracious, dignified individual whose special aristocratic air and bearing is supported by a rational approach to life.

In a word, when conditions are just right, and he understands how he must act, *Arsenicum* performs like the thoroughbred he has the potential to be.

Arsenicum album

PRINCIPAL REGIONS AFFECTED

Head   Itching scalp; dandruff; sensitive scalp (hurts to brush hair) or feels cold; **hayfever and allergy symptoms; colds with sneezing and runny nose, with acrid, watery discharge;** runny, burning eyes

Chest   **Asthma** (especially at night); various coughs and difficulties breathing; burning pains

Digestion   Cannot bear the sight or smell of food; **nausea, retching, vomiting; painful or painless diarrhea;** burning pains in stomach after eating or drinking; **ill-effects of food poisoning; food fads;** anorexia

Skin   **Itching, burning; also dry, rough, scaly, flaking;** cold sores around and canker sores in the mouth; various rashes; eczema; psoriasis; hives; impetigo

Nerves   **Great sensitivity to the external environment; high-strung;** anxiety and/or work-related concerns prevent sleep or cause **frequent waking; sleeplessness after midnight; must get up and walk around.** Dreams of day's embarrassment, cares, and vexations; of being late for an appointment or unprepared for an event; of robbers

GENERALITIES

Extreme restlessness; must be active

Chilliness, especially of extremities which can be ice cold

Sensitive to heat and comfortable only within a two- or three-degree temperature range

Exhausting cold sweats; night sweats

Burning character of pains and a number of complaints

Sudden, intense, and unbearable pains

High (nervous) energy for work or vocation

Sudden debility from overtaxing his strength

Continued.

Arsenicum album — *cont'd*

MODALITIES (< worse; > better)

Time	< Night (especially midnight to 4:00 AM); weekly or every two weeks; yearly
	> Morning
Temperature	< Cold in every form but also heat; wet weather
	> Warmth: of sun, of rooms, clothing; hot applications; but also cool air to head
Position	< Lying flat
	> Lying with head elevated; sitting up
Energy	< Inactivity
	> Working (weekend headaches); moving about (activity, walking)
Food/Drink	< Cold foods and drink; watery fruits (especially in summer); hives from fish or shellfish
	> Warm foods and drink; generally from eating and from sipping hot liquids; likes fats

GUIDING MENTAL SYMPTOMS

The perfectionist par excellence; fastidious, exacting, with extreme sensitivity to disorder, disorganization, inefficiency

Hard-working, ambitious, competitive, driven and driving individual

Controlling personality: derives security from being in charge at all times and in all situations

Irritable, fault-finding, critical and intolerant of poor performance in others, but also extremely self-critical

Obsessive/compulsive behavior; but also high self-control when he sets his mind to it

Exceptional ability to concentrate on detail

Highly represented in the creative and performing arts or in any occupation requiring meticulous attention to detail and a delicate touch

Extreme apprehension and anxiety; fears being alone; illness (hypochondriacal and despairs of recovery), accidents, death (imagines catastrophes to himself or family); contaminated food; germs and contagion; poverty; robbers; the future (waiting for some misfortune to happen)

Lachesis

The remedy *Lachesis* is derived from the venom of the Brazilian bushmaster, or surukuku, one of the most poisonous snakes found in the Western Hemisphere. The snake is remarkable for its forked tongue, and the pervasive theme in this archetypal picture is *dualism*—that is, the nature's propensity to embrace conflicting impulses, emotions, or behavioral tendencies almost simultaneously and the impact of this conflict on the psyche.

Within the *Lachesis* individual, opposing forces are constantly at war: indulgence versus restraint, arrogance versus humility, faith versus cynicism, love versus hate—each struggling to overcome the other. The split psyche is especially disconcerting to the subject himself, because he can never count on the steadiness of his own feelings and behavior. Sensing that his current mood can easily be overturned by his underlying conflicting side, he fears inconstancies and reversals he is incapable of controlling.

Complicating the picture is a struggle for supremacy among the three levels of his being: the mental, the emotional, and the sensual. *Lachesis* can be highly intellectual, displaying a fine, incisive mind that seeks to govern his feelings and behavior and to pursue a rational mode of life. Yet, he is also highly emotional, to the point of being incapable at times of relinquishing the intensity of a feeling—which possesses him, rather than he the feeling. Finally, the type can be strongly given to sensual gratification. Even if the impulse is controlled, this side of him is always making itself felt. All three irreducible forces are perpetually battling for dominion, with the patient's body as the war-torn battlefield.

Perhaps *Lachesis'* primary conflict is between his lower instincts and his higher ego. The strong animal urges seek expression, but the individual constantly suppresses them for the sake of civilized behavior and/or spiritual growth. Deprived of their natural outlet, the blocked emotions then take their toll on the individual's physical health or find vicarious outlet in unstable moods and erratic behavior. Any constitutional type may struggle with his lower instincts to attain a higher personal moral development. What distinguishes *Lachesis* is (1) the intensity of the struggle; (2) its unremitting nature (it can continue unabated throughout childhood and adult life); and (3) his awareness of it. In fact, this exceeding awareness of the underlying self (constantly reminding *Lachesis* that he is a mere step away from some unexpected reversal and that should the occasion arise, he might be tempted into some reprehensible action) threatens his peace of mind. Seemingly well-balanced individuals will confess to a fear of losing their mental balance from the pressure of excessive self-restraint or to dreading lest their energies, once released, will explode in all directions ("I'm always in conflict, always holding myself in, or holding myself back; I don't know how long I can go on this way").

The *Lachesis* nature, struggling against itself, not only eludes simple analysis but is also one on which no two observers can agree. The person who appears to some as a hurricane of energy and commotion is seen by others as a soothing summer breeze. To be sure, there is a Jekyll-and-Hyde aspect to the personality. On one hand, devotion and self-abnegation can be displayed by *Lachesis* to a very high degree. Sons and daughters will care for frail, elderly parents, caregivers for their charges, in a spirit of self-sacrifice that is wonderful to behold! The altruism of these generous souls shows little subliminal self-pity, little resentful dutifulness—still less desire for Promethean effect; they discharge their responsibilities seemingly without thought of recognition. Or, full of principle, they will act with noble renunciation in some personal matter. One woman, only moderately well-off herself, believing that the inheritance she received from her late husband more correctly belonged to his children from his first marriage, conveyed it all to them. If praised for their virtue, these individuals hardly understand what is meant, taking for granted that no other behavior is possible.

Sometimes the *Lachesis* nobility of gesture or behavior appears to others to be wild, irrational, and extravagant. Actually, it is perfectly in keeping with the type's strong impulses, which often veer off in unforeseen directions. Whether he exposes himself to slander so as to shield another, imprudently takes sides in a bitter controversy that does not directly concern him, plunges headlong into a seemingly futile altruistic venture, or in other ways displays excessive devotion toward a person or cause, there is an unaccountable, unintelligible quality to his actions. Indeed, when a high-minded *Lachesis* is on the rampage to protect, correct, reform, educate, or relieve some aspect of this sad world, the best thing others can do is to stand aside and let him rip.

This view was unwittingly echoed by a university Graduate Department head and advisor, assisting an exceptionally motivated *Lachesis* student to catapult through a rigorous four-year Ph.D. program in two and a half years. The woman was eager to accept the position of principal of a benighted (crime-ridden) high school, with the intention of reforming it through an emphasis on the performing and creative arts; hence her accelerated pace. "Speaking for myself and my colleagues," said the advisor, "I think *our* job is simply to get out of your way."

Occasionally, too, the *Lachesis* picture is encountered in the individual who, as a result of his own interminable wars of the psyche, is only too well aware of the paradoxes and weaknesses of man's nature. Having been tried by fire and emerged serene from his internal struggles and doubts, he has reached a level of compassion for humanity that ranks as true nobility of soul. Significantly, however, even when chivalrous, honorable, and generous, the constitutional type is not gentle. "Forceful" describes him better; and he will fight back if provoked or feeling threatened. The snake draws itself erect and is prepared to strike.

On the other hand, *Lachesis* can also be scheming and manipulative, capable of turning friends or family members against one another. In an abrupt reversal of her usual helping role, a family member becomes an intriguer when hostile feelings that have hitherto lain dormant suddenly become dominant. Or a student who has spent hours assisting a slower friend with her homework might one day gratuitously conspire against the latter behind her back. Her behavior is quite incomprehensible to the non-*Lachesis* victim who wonders what motivates her former best friend.

Moreover, projecting his own unpredictable mood shifts onto humanity at large, *Lachesis* tends to be suspicious of the motives and integrity of others, and fearful of betrayal. For instance, one capable young woman, trying to be ultra-successful in her profession, could talk of nothing but her colleagues' intrigue, competitiveness, and envy of her—concerns that clearly mirrored her own feelings and behavior, and which, in self-justification, she was projecting onto others.

Predictably, *Lachesis'* embracing of contrary emotions is often displayed in the love relationship. He can alternate between love and hate more suddenly and violently than any other personality type—reversing within minutes, and then just as suddenly switching back again. One could say that these opposite emotions coexist, were it not that the dominant feeling of the moment so entirely possesses the individual as to leave little room for ambivalence. Then again, perhaps these emotions are not truly opposed in *Lachesis,* since they both proceed from the same source of intense feeling. Many sages have insisted on the closeness, if not actual oneness (by virtue of being two sides of the same coin), of love and hate.

Another dichotomy is seen in the nature's capacity to be simultaneously straightforward and deceptive. He can be scrupulously truthful, at times giving the impression of an overaggressive honesty cultivated to overcome the subliminal dishonesty that chronically threatens to surface. However, he might also protest his honesty too much. His "I cannot lie," "I always tell the truth," "I never deceive," disguises a certain deviousness that sometimes catches the individual himself by surprise. His psyche operates so sinuously, so dualistically at times, that he finds himself acting underhandedly without so intending. Or, with his vivid imagination, he finds himself embellishing the truth or spinning a fictitious tale (a story worth telling is worth telling *well*).

But although *Lachesis* may resort to hypocrisy (speaking with the serpent's forked tongue), exaggeration, or mendacity, he does not deceive himself. "The serpent knows itself," is an old adage, and *Lachesis,* being in close touch with his subliminal side, has few *self*-delusions. In fact, when confronted with unpalatable truths about himself, he will, surprisingly, accept them ("Myself I may contradict; the truth I may not": Montaigne).

In the embracing of opposites, the type can combine an insensitivity of manner with an incisive awareness of the feelings and motives of others, which enables him to perceive with intense clarity the progression of others' thoughts and actions and to anticipate the events that may ensue. This lack of coordination between behavior and understanding might make him appear brusque or unheeding, as he continues his own line of thought rather than responding to another's. It eventually becomes clear, however, from his having taken effective steps to help, that even while seeming not to listen, he has intelligently understood the other's concerns ("I don't have to listen, because I always know what another is going to say").

Finally, in *Lachesis,* hotheaded impetuosity may coexist with a clear-sighted deliberation, overheated passion with cool trenchant reason; or a dictatorial decisiveness with bouts of painful irresolution. An historic (and extreme) example of these dualistic tendencies was Queen Elizabeth I of England, who was capable of both political harshness and of magnanimity and a true love for her subjects.

Her dictatorial proclivity was always vying with indecisiveness, and she employed both characteristics to wield power and retain her precarious throne. She could never decide whether or not, or whom, to marry. Advisors and retainers regularly fell in and out of her favor; her favorites, even if objects of her romantic passion, she would not hesitate to have beheaded the moment she felt them to be a threat to the State. She was undecided whether or not to take decisive steps against the Roman Catholics and Mary Queen of Scots, or what stance to take in the religious conflicts seething on all sides; whether to sign treaties with other countries or declare war on them. She shamelessly and autocratically reneged on personal commitments and in state negotiations. This vacillation drove neighboring monarchs and her advisors to distraction. But not only did her capricious instincts prove, in hindsight, to be clear-sighted and politically correct, they also contributed to her survival, both as a person and as a ruler, during the dangerous and strife-torn times in which she lived and reigned.

Altogether, this divided personality, with its erratic shifts of mood, attitude, and behavior, resembles a small sailboat tossed and buffeted in a gale and tacking first to starboard and then to port in its attempt to stay afloat and steer a course to harbor.

However contrary and ambiguous an impression *Lachesis* produces on others, few will fault him for lack of energy. Notwithstanding his internal conflicts, he exhibits such unquenchable vitality that the words that spring to mind in describing him are "intense," "overstimulated," "compulsive"—and above all, "passionate": passionate not solely in the romantic sense, but with a passion for experience, for understanding—for life itself!

His incredible energy is manifested first of all, physically, in his capacity to subsist on very little sleep. Sleep, according to the type, is a waste of time. Not only can he easily stay up into the early hours of the morning but also, after being up half the night socializing, engaging in stimulating conversation, reading, studying, or working, he is full of energy the following day and shows no sign of fatigue.

Nighttime is, in fact, when *Lachesis* really comes into his own. With heightened acumen and his creative energies reaching their peak, the mind races with an increased vigor and originality; no sooner does an idea occur to him than a number of others crowd in on him. Night is also traditionally the time when the subconscious is most aroused and the psyche most open to inspiration from the universe. Insights hit with the force of revelation—and then are expressed in bursts of creativity over which he has little control. Dostoyevsky, as purely a *Lachesis* male as ever existed, had the remedy's timetable. He would sit up nights writing in frenzied spurts of near-demonic inspiration in order to give dramatic expression to the immediacy and intensity of his insights before they evaporated with the daylight. And it was during these exhilarating all-night sessions that he was able to turn out one major novel every two years.

Even in everyday life, the vital temperament can be observed; the more *Lachesis* does the more energy he generates. He may accomplish so much on the job that it takes three persons to fill his position when he leaves or retires. He is never fatigued, never slows down, and since he can get along for long periods with minimal sleep, his days seem to contain more hours than other people's do. A familiar figure, for example, is the *Lachesis* school or university teacher who not only adores her work but also never wearies of the same subject, every year bringing to it a freshness drawn from her own unabated enthusiasm. She has so much to say that she can never finish the class on time. If she has thirty tests to grade, they are all given back the next morning. Term papers are corrected with equal alacrity, the perceptive comments on every page revealing that hers was no perfunctory reading. She will have stayed up all night reading and correcting them, also preparing for class. But in school the next day she is as full of vitality as ever, showing no sign of sleeplessness and with seemingly unlimited attention to give to even the most demanding student. Watching *Lachesis* operate at full throttle, the observer can only wonder where all that energy comes from.

Nor does this type require a supportive environment to function productively. His vitality remains undiminished in the face of adversity ("I feel as if I've been in combat all year, but I'm feeling great anyway"). At times it appears as if the more trying the circumstances, the higher he soars in a kind of manic reaction to stress. It is significant that *Lachesis* Harriet Beecher Stowe wrote her famous antislavery novel, *Uncle Tom's Cabin,* under conditions of extreme hardship—sickness, financial stringency, emotional trials—when she was only able to work at night, after having discharged her manifold family and household obligations. She claimed that the story came to her "almost as a tangible vision" and that it was not merely inspired, but "written by God" (in a *Lachesis* exalted, trancelike state?). Certainly, her subsequent nine novels, written under relatively easy conditions after *Uncle Tom's Cabin* had made her fortune and reputation, were unremarkable. Likewise, Dostoyevsky, reacting to the stress of poverty and epilepsy and working under the deadlines of his serialized fiction, proved himself to work best under extreme pressure.

This, to be sure, is part of *Lachesis'* problem. His energy is so plentiful, his vitality so strong, that at times he cannot handle it constructively, cannot direct it so as to avoid harming himself. When his intensity, vigor, and fertile mind are properly channeled, his creative output is unsurpassed. But, by virtue of being something of a force of nature, his energies are not always easy to channel. Also, sometimes he falls short of true distinction because his creativity, like his energy, is chaotic. By virtue of his inspiration erupting in sporadic bursts, the quality of his performance is uneven.

The *Lachesis* vitality exhibits one additional and quite unique feature. It is so plentiful, so powerful, that in its superfluity it spills over and has a capacity to infect others. A person can feel tired, drained, or discouraged at the end of a long day, but after a short time in the presence of this constitutional type, he begins to come alive and feels vibrant and alert—quite ready to start the day anew.

In his heightened assertion of life and determination to experience it to the fullest, *Lachesis* is ever seeking some cause, strong belief, intense relationship, or all-engrossing artistic or professional commitment. If he does not find an outlet in one of these, his over-abundant vitality might turn for stimulation to an addiction: alcohol, coffee, gambling, shopping sprees, food, or other forms of bingeing.

The sexual drive is usually strong in both men and women, and without the calming effect of a normal sex life, they may visibly suffer. In biblical and mythical tradition the serpent symbolizes both sexuality *and* the higher realms of knowledge (including the urge to learn and grow through tasting life). By thus containing within itself the seed of spiritual development, sex to the dualistic *Lachesis* mind might take on the attributes of religion, and he will seek in sexual passion the mystery and revelatory fervor traditionally provided by religion. Therefore, although *Lachesis* can be a philanderer, he may antithetically be the most devoted and loyal of spouses, throughout the whole of his married life directing all the intensity of his sexual nature toward one woman. One man claimed that in all the years of married life, he had never for one single moment regretted marrying his wife. In fact, he woke up every morning and went to bed every night "thanking God for the blessing of a good marriage." This was very touching and obviously true, as his wife was like a religion to him. But he was also very possessive of her, not liking her even to say a good word about another man.

The picture of single-minded devotion is even more prevalent in the woman. She can be passionately in love with her partner for life, for all that he may be an alcoholic or in other ways an erring mate. Yet she herself is not always easy to live with, being often unduly possessive and subject to unfounded jealousy. She is suspicious of every letter or telephone call her partner receives and fears that he is deceiving her every time he comes home late. Even if she does not cross-examine him or make a scene, she still nurses a gnawing and unrelenting dread of betrayal that allows her no peace of mind. And if she learns that she has been spurned or betrayed, the humility and selflessness of love quickly turn into their opposites—into unbearable humiliation and outraged pride—at which times she is not wholly responsible for her behavior. The injured *Lachesis* might act on violent impulse, heedless of the consequences. (Naturally, this jealousy or possessiveness is by no means limited to the object of sexual or romantic love but can extend to friends and family.)

Barring the ever-present possibility of an unpredictable about-face when he feels threatened, *Lachesis* himself is loyal, and strongly stresses this quality in personal relations. Once he chooses a friend, partner, or protégé, he will strive unstintingly to preserve the relationship and benefit the other. Moreover, with his capacity to go straight to the heart and penetrate another's psyche and feelings, he knows exactly what to say and how to behave to establish a strong connection—in this way attracting those fervent friendships and eliciting those intense loyalties that he is forever seeking. However, at times he is likely to grow excessively demanding—to the point (since others may not possess his emotional energy) of endangering a relationship. Fearing the loss of a friend or loved one, he coils himself around that person, thereby forcing the other to seek an escape from *Lachesis'* too-heavy and enveloping emotions—and ultimately bringing about that which this type fears most. In short, the type's loyalty and affection is, at its source, often an excess of devotion and self-sacrifice, which has a way of backfiring negatively in a world that is not framed for so much intensity.

Lachesis, then, is intrinsically of a devotional nature. If of a religious bent, the Deity to him is an almost concrete presence with whom he communicates on terms of familiarity. When asked if he shares his problems with others or keeps them to himself, more often than other constitutional types, he will reply, "I do neither. I tell them to God and need no one else"; or words to that effect. Indeed, his fortitude in ill-health and other trials frequently issues from this unshakable faith; he is sustained by the conviction that the Lord will provide him with the necessary strength.

However, the salient point here is that this is the individual who requires constant grist for his high-powered emotional mill. If there is insufficient religious faith in his personal life, he finds an outlet for his devotional needs in some alternate set of convictions. For example, Sigmund Freud held in horror anything carrying the taint of religion, but its place in his thinking was taken by sexuality, and he expounded his views with a dogmatism that allowed no deviation from the true doctrine. In fact, his heavily sexual psychology, with its basic premise that religion and all cultural and artistic activity are largely sublimations of sexual neuroses or repressed sexuality, carries a truly *Lachesis* coloration. Additionally, Freud exhibited the type's insistence on personal loyalty or solidarity, displaying anger or indignation if a disciple (notably Carl Jung) strayed from the true path and branched out on his own.

Noteworthy in this connection is the compelling quality of *Lachesis'* beliefs. He can be so forcibly struck by some particular conviction as to reject even the possibility of a dissenting one. He forgets to take into account that different people are ready for different revelations at different times in their lives or that they may espouse their own particular philosophies and therefore be less receptive to another's. His own vision *must* be, always *has been,* and, prophetically, always *will* be true for all mankind, and he proceeds to apply it to humanity in a Procrustean manner. Dostoyevsky, as well as Freud, has already been mentioned as typifying the *Lachesis* mentality. Both men displayed that intensity of feeling and conviction that amounts virtually to a revelation; both saw themselves as prophets, and did, in truth, venture into previously unexplored regions of the soul. The works of both exhibit the sort of intellectual seductiveness and compelling subjective style typical of *Lachesis*—leading the reader to believe that the theories propounded embrace the whole truth and not just a segment of it. Thus, the *Lachesis* intellect is distinguished not so much by breadth of vision (as with *Sulphur*), but rather by its depth and intensity.

But with his bifurcated mind, *Lachesis* is also (at times simultaneously) subject to doubts and wavering convictions. Sensing two opposing forces in himself, he easily becomes aware of the duality, and consequent neutrality, of all phenomena. With his proclivity for constantly reexamining his own motives, he might indulge in a circular and psychologically debilitating self-analysis, which leads to motives, actions, and feelings taking on the attributes of their opposites: Was an act of charity prompted by true kindness or a desire for world approval? Was some renunciation a sincere expression of noble generosity or prompted by secret pride? This circular analysis is symbolized in the image of the snake eating its own tail.

Moral turmoil, intellectual conflict, and loss of faith are hardly specific to any one constitutional type. But when individuals begin to question their religion or vocation; experience soul-searing doubts about their ideals, marriage, or personal development; and project their own inner conflicts onto the world at large, the serpent mentality may be suspected. Even basically non-*Lachesis* constitutional types may require the remedy when undergoing some profound disillusionment, self-examination, or reassessment during their midlife passage.

Lachesis' interminable internal struggles are perhaps one reason why the appearance of physical discharges such as tears, coryzas, nosebleeds, even urination and bowel movements (conceivably serving as surrogate outlets for the blocked instincts and emotions) markedly ameliorates a number of ailments and complaints. This particular modality is by far most commonly encountered in the relief accorded a woman by her menstrual period. Weepiness, touchiness, despondency, increased irritability or unaccountable behavior ("I am not myself before my period," a woman will say. "I seem to go crazy and completely lose control! My whole personality changes. I become aggressive with my husband, tyrannical with the children, and abusive if things aren't going my way")—all disappear as if by magic once the flow sets in. And the natural corollary to this "better from physical discharges" picture is the emergence of ailments and undesirable physical symptoms, of violent mood swings or unpredictable behavior, during menopause.

Just as *Lachesis* feels better from physical discharges, so this individual finds substantial relief in mental discharges—specifically, words. Instincts and emotions denied a normal physical expression will often find a surrogate expression in excessive verbosity. An unending flow of words is one of the classic signs of an emotionally unfulfilled or creatively thwarted personality. This characteristic is especially pronounced in the woman, probably because up until recently her sexual and creative energies have been more suppressed than those of men. She can virtually talk (or write) herself out of a strong anger or depression. Once all is verbalized, a measure of calm or hope returns. Thus, although use of the masculine pronoun has been preserved throughout this analysis, the *Lachesis* picture (perhaps for the reason just mentioned) is definitely encountered more frequently in women than in men.

The word "loquacious" applies to Lachesis more than to any other type. The woman frequently expresses her thoughts in a rush of words, as if hurrying to catch up with her thoughts before they slip away. Once started, she cannot control her pace, cannot slow down—to the point that sometimes the tongue moves quicker than the ear can catch. Additionally, once launched into speech, it is hard for her to stop. When a subject is of particular interest to her, there is no arresting the flow of words and their attached associations, with one idea breeding another. A simple question is likely to provoke a torrent of explanations or a stream of digressions in reply. She might also exhibit a tendency to leave sentences uncompleted. Like the snake's tongue that darts from one side to another, the mind darts from thought to thought in disconnected phrases. A word in the preceding sentence reminds her of another idea, and she strikes off on a new tangent, then may or may not return to conclude the initial thought. Occasionally, she gets lost in her multiple threads of dangling thoughts and saltations from one subject to another and will draw herself up, saying, "Now where was I? What was I saying?"

Sometimes, exhilarated by conversation, the mind works so fast, with the tongue following so closely behind, that anticipating another's train of thought, *Lachesis* jumps in to complete a sentence for him—literally taking the words out of his mouth. The interjected word or phrase may be perceptive and remarkably accurate, but the other still feels like crying out, "Let me say it myself, for Heaven's sake!" Furthermore, an uncontrolled tongue that leaves nothing *un*-said also indicates the type. But then the woman might claim that the words are not deliberate, that they escape of their own accord. She fights this tendency, but gratuitously tactless or cutting remarks slip out in unguarded moments ("Something just *drives* me. I can't *not* say what I have the urge to say. I actually have *no* control"). Loss of control in any sphere is a familiar *Lachesis* confession.

Conversely, individuals of either sex can use language with dramatic effect. *Lachesis* is the orator who stirs up an audience with his emotionally charged language, the preacher who can penetrate straight to the hearts of his listeners, the lecturer whose delivery carries a note of ecstasy—or merely the person who conveys passionate conviction.

Finally, a laconic type also exists, although less easily recognized than the voluble one. This is the person (more often a male) who, concealing an incisive mind, silently takes in everything around him—only periodically throwing out a trenchant or cutting remark. Like the ever-watchful snake, he lies quietly coiled, but ready to strike. Pith and economy of expression and the ability to use few words with keen penetration (with the sharpness of the serpent's tooth) are all a part of the *Lachesis* picture.

At times a curious aura of impersonality emanates from the *Lachesis* individual, as though on some emotional level hardships do not affect him as they do others. The trials and tribulations he recounts may be intellectually intriguing but do not rend the heart. He does not elicit pity because he does not ask for it. It is not that he is insensitive to emotional trauma; on the contrary, he suffers deeply and often pays a heavy physical or mental price for wounds of the past. But he appears to maintain a distance between himself and his troubles, displaying a philosophical acceptance of the part he is fated to play in the ebbs and flows of this earthly existence. Such acceptance of trials and tragedy (as if he were an observer in a drama larger than himself) is partly what gives him the capacity to endure hardship and adversity with uncommon valor.

An impersonal approach to one's difficulties favors a humorous attitude, and, notwithstanding the misfortune of a given situation, in

Lachesis a touch of the ridiculous is often blended with the distressing. Sometimes the individual himself encourages this impression by emphasizing the comic side of his hardships. He is quick to extract the ridiculous from harrowing experiences—perhaps deliberately creating a distance between himself and his mishaps by recounting the series of absurd misadventures and bizarre calamities that seem to shadow him at every turn. Or perhaps in his sensitive pride he is ensuring that others are laughing *with* and not *at* him. Thus, the humorist whose laconic wit or whose one quip after another offers a running commentary on everyday life, might well be a *Lachesis*. Often, however, one senses beneath the surface that this person has in some way been defeated by life; that fate has conferred on him more than his fair share of hardships, and for him wit is the only outlet from an intolerable or unalterably tragic situation. It is hardly surprising, then, that *Lachesis* should harbor a shadow side to his infectious vitality. For all his surface love of the absurd, for all his easily exhilarated mood and his frequently exalted state, this is the individual who will at times effect a complete withdrawal from the world, with no desire to mix with it, and will display the hopelessness, despair, and loathing of life of a true manic-depressive. After all, are not the humorous and tragic outlooks complementary expressions of a profoundly felt meaninglessness and futility of all worldly matters?

Much *Lachesis* disharmony thus arises from the conflict between an individual's opposing selves. Within the divided psyche, overstimulation and overgratification compete with moral or intellectual restraint, skepticism competes with devotion, emotion with reason, laughter with despair. The warring factions are not easily reconciled, and the torn, conflicted personality visibly struggles as he seeks a oneness in himself—some "wholeness" within which to resolve, or at least reconcile, the clashes of his dualistic nature. True harmony will elude him, however, until his devotional nature finds firm ground to rest on in a strong faith, in a worthy dedication to a person or a cause, or in an artistic discipline providing him with a higher spiritual or mental integration. Only then will the different sides of his nature, each seeking supremacy, no longer feel in perpetual strife, but can coexist in a more peaceful, albeit at times still precarious, state of truce.

Lachesis

PRINCIPAL REGIONS AFFECTED

Head	Throbbing, burning, pulsating pains, extending into eyes, cannot maintain focus; **waves of pain; sun headaches;** migraines usually left-sided
Throat	Left-sided pain, sometimes with stitching into ears and/or **pain on empty swallowing; sensation of lump in throat;** spasms, constriction, as of suffocation
Cardiovascular	Palpitations; **constricted feeling in chest;** irregular beats; **sepsis; varicose veins; tendency to bleed excessively**
Digestion	Chokes on food when eating fast, food bingeing
Female	Fibroids; ovarian pain and/or cysts (left-sided); high sexual energy; various menstrual **complaints: premenstrual symptoms,** with sadness, irritability, heat (wants to throw off clothing), **headaches; interrupted flow;** excessive bleeding; aggravation of symptoms after menses ceases; **menopausal complaints: hot flashes,** palpitations (with fainting spells), excessive bleeding, uncontrolled emotions
Skin	Tight and shiny, or **mottled, livid, bluish-purple, or blue-black** swellings; ulcerations and infections

GENERALITIES

Predominantly a female remedy

Individual is warm-blooded and generates much internal heat

Flushes of heat to head or over entire body

Unstable temperature with partial chills and sweats

Energy can be so plentiful as to be chaotic, uncontrolled—bouncing off the walls

Energy alternates with collapse and complete inertia—even withdrawal from the world

Constricted feeling around the neck

Feelings of suffocation come on during sleep; wakens from inability to breathe

Sudden starting when falling asleep; sleepy, yet cannot sleep

Complaints usually left-sided or moving from left to right

Continued.

Lachesis—cont'd

MODALITIES (< worse; > better)

Time	< Morning, upon awakening; after sleep (anytime of day); yearly, especially springtime
	> **Night: wide awake at bedtime; mental labor best performed at night**
Temperature	< Heat: sun, warm room, clothes, hot bathing; spring, summer; cloudy weather
	> Cold: air, bathing, seasons
Food/Drink	< Hot drinks (except when sore throat); **alcohol;** coffee
	> Cold drinks; **swallowing solid foods;** hot drinks (with a sore throat); fruit and fruit juices
Other	< **Sleep; individual sleeps into aggravation, or ailments come on during sleep**
	> **Discharges and free secretions:** tears, urine, bowel movements, perspiration; **menses:** amelioration of all symptoms as soon as flow sets in
	< Slightest touch; **pressure of clothes, especially around the neck, but also other parts of the body**
	> **Hard pressure**
	< **Suppression of emotions**

GUIDING MENTAL SYMPTOMS

Vital, intense, passionate nature

Vivid imagination; witty, sharp-tongued

Loquacity; jumps from one subject to another; leaves sentences unfinished

Intense emotionalism; suspicion, jealousy, unpredictable behavior

Internal conflicts; the higher nature combatting the lower instincts

Dislikes feeling pressured, yet operates well under extreme pressure and himself generates pressured situations

Effects of severe trauma: tragic losses, heartbreak, bizarre calamities (and generally being dealt a difficult hand in life)

Middle age crises of women

Manic-depressive picture

Fears snakes, being poisoned, loss of reason; loss of faith or a life meaning

Silica

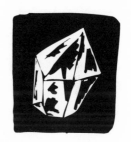

The remedy *Silica* is prepared from silicon dioxide, a whitish or colorless granular mineral distributed abundantly in the earth either in its pure crystalline form or as quartz, flint, or sand.

The archetypal picture of this constitutional type is not easy to grasp. Just as a piece of cut crystal reflects innumerable facets even as it draws the eye inward into its depths, so is the often inwardly directed *Silica* nature, when closely examined, seen to harbor numerous subtly varying and sometimes contrasting aspects. Nevertheless, in the following pages an attempt will be made to present a clear and cohesive analysis of the *Silica* personality.

Think of a grain of quartz sand and of how long and slow the process is that brought it to its present (and now unchanging) form. On the physical level, this process is reflected in the *Silica* picture of slow growth and chronicity. The body has a tendency to form cysts, nodes, fatty and fibrous tumors that grow slowly and, once formed, are there to stay; and chronicity is the hallmark of ear or sinus infections, lingering respiratory ailments, and various skin affections. Slow healing and weak recuperative powers are exemplified in the unending suppuration of minor cuts and fistulas; in infections from splinters; in old wounds that have never healed properly and old scars that still ache; in boils and abscesses that refuse to come to a head; in recurring felons, hangnails, and cracks in the skin; in pimples and crusty eruptions that peel off only to return, and so on. Moreover, because of a delicate physique, *Silica* might possess a low vitality. For instance, he produces so little animal warmth that he has to wear socks in bed at night and keep his head well-wrapped during the day—while exposure to drafts and air-conditioning, or especially getting chilled after being overheated, is near-lethal. As a result, he might spend so much energy trying, in this or other ways, to acclimatize to his physical environment that little time is left for a full, active life.

Slow growth and chronicity patterns are likewise encountered in the mental-emotional sphere. Often *Silica* develops and matures slowly. He is late passing through the normal human rites of passage: integrating socially, securing a steady job, marrying, assuming the responsibilities of parenthood, finding his true calling. For instance, the eternal student is often a *Silica*. Despite taking course after course in his chosen field and amassing far more credits than are requisite for the degree, he postpones taking that final examination or writing that final obligatory paper or in other ways completing his studies. In the meantime, he continues to haunt the university libraries year after year, unable to muster the energy or resolve to embark on a profession. Or, in a variation on this theme, he is the university or professional-school graduate with good intellectual capacities who, despite a good academic record—despite years of attending postgraduate conferences, specialized training courses, and in other ways girding for action—postpones taking his place among the shakers and movers of the world. Instead, he may decide to take time off (which can amount to years) before he eventually settles into a serious professional commitment commensurate with his abilities. In the meantime, however, he pursues his own quiet interests and a modest existence far more contentedly than others embark on an active and affluent existence.

At times *Silica*'s slowness to recuperate assumes the form of brain fatigue. This is the individual who has never been well since some strenuous or prolonged mental exertion—never mind that the effort occurred many months earlier. Even without the excuse of uncommon exertion, followed by collapse, his mental stamina can be poor and he is easily tired by efforts of memory or concentration. Also rising from the type's "chronicity" mode is his difficulty terminating a project: whether a building contractor his house, a woman the dress she is sewing, an artist his or her painting. Ninety or ninety-five percent of the task gets accomplished, but then he hangs on to the last five percent, unable to relinquish it. One *Silica* scholar complained to his homoeopath of being unable to send out his book (long overdue) for publication. When questioned why this should be, he admitted to having trouble finishing the concluding chapter. "I've been writing it for more than six months, but it keeps getting longer and longer. I am up to page seventy-five, and still there is no end in sight. I know I shouldn't touch it. It's perfect as it is, and I wish I could stop! But something is preventing me from letting go." Such a loud call for *Silica* could not be ignored, and the medicine was prescribed. Shortly thereafter, the offending chapter (only eighty pages long!) was completed.

Silica's slow growth, weakened mental stamina, and chronicity do not preclude competence, purpose, and an ability to work hard and well. However, like flint—an inert stone that yields a spark only when struck or abraded—this individual may require some catalyst (such as the homoeopathic remedy) to ignite the spark that stimulates accomplishment or hastens an unfinished project to completion.

Finally, because a slow, gradual growth characterizes his style and tempo, whatever his age or intellectual capacities, *Silica* can appear callow and somewhat naive. This last characteristic, together with the type's chirpiness, contentment, and quiet charm, has been captured by Charles Dickens in the person of Herbert Pocket in *Great Expectations*—the "pale young gentleman of slight build . . . with a figure that looked as if it would always be light and young . . . [who yet] had a certain languor about him in the midst of his spirits and briskness that did not seem indicative of natural strength . . . [and who possessed, also, an air of] wonderful hopefulness, that at the same time whispered to me that he would never be successful or rich."

"Want of grit" is a classic phrase applied to *Silica*—and, in certain respects, justly so. The type might well lack enterprise, daring, mettle, pluck—in a word, the very "sand" from which the remedy derives. The association between courage and sand is a commonplace in American folklore, and in Mark Twain's novel *Huckleberry Finn,* fourteen-year-old Huck admires the spunk and fire of Mary Jane Wilks in the following words: "Pray for me! I reckon if she knowed me she'd take a job that was more nearer her size. But I bet she done it, just the same. . . . She had the grit to pray for Judas if she took the notion. . . . You may say what you want to, but in my opinion she had more sand in her than any girl I ever see; in my opinion she was just full of *sand.*"

Lacking nerve, a *Silica* might refuse to undertake a venture well within his powers. Or, if he does undertake it, he tests out every step before venturing on the next, carefully rationing out his energies precisely according to what he judges he can or cannot accomplish. In so doing, he resembles a person at the foot of a tall ladder: if he raises his sights too high, he becomes frightened by the height and by the effort required to make the ascent, but if he looks up only as far as the next step (that is, is allowed to proceed at his own deliberate pace), he will eventually reach the top. A case in point was the *Silica* author who wrote an excellent book on a particular social issue. It had started out as a five-page article in an obscure journal and was followed by subsequent short articles, which found their way into similarly obscure publications, until his literary output eventually grew into a sizable volume. "Had I been asked to write a book from the outset," he confessed, "I never would have dared attempt it."

Another common manifestation of *Silica*'s want of grit is a fear of performing in public, with its accompanying anticipatory dreads. The clergyman fears delivering his sermon, the professor his lecture, the attorney addressing the court, the student giving an oral report, the seasoned actor or musician going on stage. This anticipatory dread commences long in advance of the event itself and is to be distinguished from the "jitters" just before a performance or from real stage fright. When actually put to the test, *Silica* acquits himself creditably and his performance goes off well.

A natural corollary to his overall timidity is *Silica*'s tendency to underrate his abilities. A telling instance of this self-underestimation was encountered in one of two scholars, both of whom had published serious articles in their respective fields. These being rather specialized and esoteric, neither man had received much recognition, but the *Silica* author at once decided that his article, although not without merit, was unpalatable. "It is hardly surprising that it went unnoticed," he remarked. "Who wants to read a ponderous and dull work in which every phrase has the specific gravity of lead?" The *Sulphur/Lycopodium* author, in contrast, while admitting that his article was suffering the fate of a note in a bottle cast into the Atlantic (he fell in love with this simile and repeated it on every possible occasion), remained quite unperturbed. "No fear," he said. "This is a first-class piece of scholarship, and if it is above most people's heads—Well, they'll just have to stretch their minds a little. In due course it will be read by those who can appreciate it."

Generally speaking, confronting a new task, *Silica* hesitates, feels overwhelmed, bemoans his insufficiency ("I always fear that I'm slipping and won't be able to perform; yet I manage well enough. But the fact that I manage 'well enough,' makes others think me more capable than I am; and this leaves me even more insecure"). Nevertheless, he will apply himself conscientiously—and ultimately produces results where another, seemingly more promising, merely produces excuses, justifications, and expressions of regret for failing to perform. This is one scenario. However, there is also a contrasting one. Because he remains convinced of his (often imaginary) incompetence and lacks nerve, he might refuse to shoulder responsibilities or attempt to distinguish himself in a way easily within his capacity. In fact, he appears to be as apprehensive of attracting the world's notice to himself as other types are of being ignored.

It is perhaps this very timidity, combined with his frequently low social energy that contributes to *Silica*'s fundamentally non-aggressive disposition. Conflict, pugnacity, contention, confrontation all require effort, which he would rather avoid. Indeed, a large portion of his life is devoted to steering clear of offense or friction and, with time, he grows expert at retiring from a scene that is not perfectly attuned to his sensibilities and at going his own independent way. Carried a step further, he might be so averse to contention as to refuse to defend his position and would rather be considered wrong than take the trouble to prove himself correct. In his professional life he might so lack the entrepreneurial mentality that he lets others seek out opportunities and collar the more interesting (and demanding) jobs—at times even allowing them to usurp a position that rightfully belongs to him. One *Silica* with somewhat hermit tendencies volunteered that he had never accomplished much of significance in life because he expended so much energy working out his various fears and timidities, or protecting himself from being imposed on, that no time remained for anything else ("I have spent most of my life in hiding").

Silica may lack the fire and spunk of Mary Jane Wilks; he won't be one to set the pond on fire. Yet he is not without his own more subtle form of courage: the quiet, fine-spun courage that shows itself where matters of principle and conscience are at stake. Here he reveals unexpected firmness and moral resolve. There was no want of grit in Ralph Waldo Emerson, the nineteenth century New England sage who in his constitutional picture exhibits a strong *Silica* vein. Emerson may have been perhaps a bit thin-blooded in his natural asceticism and want of animal vitality—seemingly too refined for intimate contact with the world. A relentless exponent of self-sufficiency and the infinitude of the individual, he articulated his reclusive *Silica* instincts as follows: "Man is insular and cannot be touched. Every man is an infinitely repellent orb, and holds his individual being on that condition . . . Most persons whom I see in my own house, I see across a gulf! I cannot go to them nor they to me." However, his aloofness was tempered by a courageous humanitarianism that made him an early and outspoken champion of the anti-slavery cause, when the rest of New England's intellectual class had not yet squarely confronted this issue—at that time controversial, bitter, even dangerous.

Additional properties of the crystalline rock are hardness and inflexibility; once *formed* as quartz, flint, sand, or pure crystal, it does not change. These two properties find their mental counterparts in the constitutional type's obduracy, persistence, and tenacity. *Silica* appears to be mild, even malleable; he will not argue, might even appear to acquiesce, but there is an unyielding side to his nature. He will not be influenced on matters either great or small—and is always able to muster sufficient energy to resist pressure and defend his right to his own ideas. And because he is persistent, he often induces others to deal with him on his own terms.

Obduracy and tenacity will sometimes cause *Silica* to become rigid in his opinions. He knows what he knows and has no desire to think differently. It is not so much a narrowness of outlook, nor that he is opinionated—still less is he intolerant by nature; but he is dismissive of matters not to his taste or in perfect tune with his psyche. He is perfectly prepared to grant that some idea may be of intrinsic value and is important to others, but it is not for him—and therefore not worthy of his perusal. And at times his dismissiveness hardens into fixed ideas. Whether it is a conviction of inability to perform or succeed at a job, his notions about diet and health regimens, or judgments of books or people, his opinion will not be shaken—evidence to the contrary notwithstanding.

Silica's inflexibility, however, is a decided strength when it translates into firmness where matters of principle or moral issues are concerned. Here (as was observed in Emerson) the nature is uncompromising, and even the mildest person will not be pressured into acting in violation of his convictions or beliefs. For all his appearance of frailty, *Silica* is as unyielding as crystal, which might eventually break under pressure but will never bend.

Another facet of the *Silica* mentality that could be viewed as hardness (in the sense of lack of feeling or an ungiving attitude) is his ability to distance himself from people and their problems, and his highly developed self-protective techniques against imposition. If his strength or peace of mind is threatened, he quietly withdraws from the scene, claiming illness or fatigue. One young woman, sincerely attached to an ailing grandmother, had to give up caring for her (thus appearing callously to shirk her share of the responsibility) because after pouring all her strength into the task undertaken, she would invariably develop a headache. Another *Silica* might collapse after trying to hold his own in a friction-full family situation. Thereafter, although fond of his home and fearful of leaving it, he forces himself to move out of the parental nest and live alone rather than become too deeply enmeshed in family dynamics. While some might view this dissociating attitude as a form of hardness of the heart, it is in reality the unaggressive person's way of guarding against emotional trauma or exploitation. *Silica* eschews challenges that are physically and psychologically draining precisely because he is aware of the limits of his strength and endurance and has learned how to conserve his energy; also because he knows that, being thoroughly reliable, once he commits to a task he does not spare himself.

For *Silica* is nothing if not conscientious. Indeed, in an attempt to perform well the type can carry conscientiousness to an extreme. Where *Arsenicum* can spend several hours packing and repacking a suitcase until everything is "just right," *Silica* can spend a week. Or an amateur carpenter might well spend days to fix a leaking faucet—while to install a door or hang a pegboard in the kitchen takes weeks. This ultraconscientiousness over small matters is caricatured in the *Peanuts* cartoon strip depicting Snoopy (that most *Phosphorus* of canines and born actor) in his current role as a *Silica* author, sitting at his typewriter on the roof of his doghouse, writing the first sentence of the opening chapter of his "great American novel." He begins the first sentence with "It"; then he thinks a while and changes it to "When." Then he tears up the page and starts again with "The." In the final panel he tells himself with beaming satisfaction, "A good writer will sometimes search for hours for just the right word."

Finally, lending itself to the theme of hardness is *Silica*'s undeniable critical streak. Not only is he discriminative and strictly selective in his judgment of people, he also possesses high standards. If others do not live up to his ideas, he dismisses them. But if he is critical of others, he is even harder on himself. In fact, his self-criticism and the demands he makes on himself introduce the final facet of crystal to be examined: its pure, clear transparency—suggestive of the human *Silica*'s delicacy, refinement, and particular form of mental clarity.

The type is often physically delicate. He is subject to inner and outer tremblings, startles easily from noise, touch, or in his sleep and is sensitive to many of the harsh physical aspects of our world. The overrefined princess in the fairy tale who could not sleep for the pea under her six mattresses ("I scarcely closed my eyes. Goodness knows what was in my bed! I lay upon something so hard that I am black and blue all over!") must have been a *Silica*.

More significantly, however, he exhibits a refinement of behavior, tastes, understanding. As a rule, he is unassuming, free from self-importance or the desire for display. If ambitious, he is quietly so, accomplishing things first and talking about them later—if at all. Lack of ostentation, a reluctance to thrust himself forward, a preference for remaining in the background—even his lack of self-confidence—all proceed, at least in part, from his refined tastes and high standards. He is fully aware of what it takes to deliver a superior address, give a superior performance, produce a worthy piece of scholarship or art—and fears lest he fall short. Additionally, there is true delicacy in his considerateness of others' feelings and wishes and in his manner of conducting himself so as not to make waves. He is stable in family relations and reliable in friendship, does not take advantage of those who love him, and arrogance seldom characterizes the type. That he possesses integrity is exemplified in the way he will not embellish on reality and is one of the few constitutional types that will not accept exaggerated praise or will disclaim praise if unearned (*Sepia* and *Natrum muriaticum* are the others). Being without guile, he can be depended on meaning what he says. And that which is even more rare, he is principled without being self-righteous.

Crystal has traditionally been associated with superior mental clarity, as attested to by the phrases "thoughts as clear as crystal" or some idea being "crystal clear"; and *Silica*'s clear thinking is reflected in fair-mindedness—especially (and this despite his inherently critical nature) where humanity is concerned. He may lack the warmth of *Phosphorus* or the uncritical sympathy of *Pulsatilla,* but he judges people with discernment as well as discrimination. He accurately assesses others' intellectual capacities and moral potential, easily detects pretense and sees through flattery, and correctly gauges the extent of his influence over others. *Silica* is the sentinel who, locked largely within his own thoughts, turns on the world a cautious, critical eye. Sensing, however, that criticism deals only in shadows and wishing to partake of the light of magnanimity—and, above all, being aware of how hard it is for every human being to lead a truly moral existence—he makes a concerted effort to be not only fair but also generous in his judgment.

A final characteristic, related to mental clarity, and with which crystal has traditionally been associated, is clairvoyance. (Recall the almost obligatory crystal ball of the gypsy fortune-teller.) Just as a piece of cut crystal reveals to the eye more than one dimension in its depths, so a *Silica* individual senses dimensions other than those usually ascribed to the physical world. Like *Phosphorus,* the type is no stranger to entities visiting from the spirit world, to visionary or prophetic dreams, to out-of-body or other paranormal experiences.

In conclusion, the type may be apprehensive of venturing into the larger world; he might choose to live and function within a rela-

tively confined and narrow space. But within these partially constitutional, partially self-imposed confines, one can bank on a principled fairness and a love of truth governing his actions and reactions.
Herein lies the strength and virtue of the often retiring, sometimes
aloof, *Silica* personality.

Silica

PRINCIPAL REGIONS AFFECTED

Head	Pain begins at the occiput, spreads over the head, and settles over the eyes; profuse sweating of the head, especially at night; affections of the **eustachian tubes,** lachrymal ducts, nasal septum, and **sinus cavities**
Throat	Cold settles in the throat, with stinging, sticking, splinterlike pains
Digestion	**Malnutrition, emaciation from want of appetite or poor assimilation of food;** constipation, with "bashful stool" (stool recedes after being partially expelled); rectal fistulas
Glands	**Hard, swollen, or enlarged** (cervical, parotid, axillary, inguinal, etc.)
Female	Breast abscesses and fistulas, also hard lumps; mastitis of nursing mothers; constipation around menses; acrid, itchy vaginal discharges; abscesses and cysts in genital area
Skin	**Slow to heal; every injury festers, suppurates, or ulcerates;** tendency to form boils, cysts, fatty tumors, abscesses on any part of the body; remedy promotes expulsion of foreign bodies, such as splinters, from the tissues; profuse, sour-smelling (and at times offensive) night sweats; offensive perspiration of feet; ingrown toenails

GENERALITIES

Slow healing or recovery pattern

Low energy, easily exhausted; exertion followed by collapse

Coldness before an attack of illness

Sensitive to nervous excitement, light, noise, jarrings to spine, pain or physical discomfort

Sleeplessness with hot head and sudden starting in sleep; somnambulism

Dreams of floods, fire, earthquakes, and other catastrophes

Ill-effects of vaccination

MODALITIES (< worse; > better)

Time   < New moon; secondarily, full moon

Temperature   < Cold in every form: air, drafts, uncovering any part of
                    the body; cold bathing, raw dampness, air-conditioning;
                    suppressed perspiration (i.e., cold bathing after being
                    heated)

                  > Warmth: applications, clothing (especially wrapping up
                    head and keeping sinus area warm)

Food/Drink   < Milk (can cause cramping and diarrhea); alcohol

GUIDING MENTAL SYMPTOMS

Delicacy of feelings and mental refinement

Fair-minded, detached; tries to maintain rectitude and emotional
   equanimity

An unassuming, mild, shy, or retiring manner, but underlying is a firm,
   unyielding, intractable disposition

Set in his opinions, with fixed ideas

Proceeds in life at his own pace

Fear of failure, of performing in public, of taking risks; of going out into
   the world to seek his fortune

Nux vomica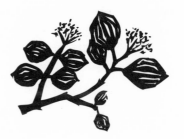

T his homoeopathic remedy, made from the potentized seed of the *Strychnos nux vomica* or poison nut (thus a form of strychnine) and affecting every part and aspect of the human economy, illustrates the old adage that the strongest poisons make the best medicines (*Ubi virus, ibi virtus*). Even more: the type of physical and mental symptoms elicited during the homoeopathic "provings" of the medicine and cured in clinical practice suggest that the pace and stresses of contemporary civilized life, together with its various stimuli, contribute to the *Nux vomica* diathesis. Few persons can avoid displaying at least traces of this personality picture and of requiring the remedy at some point in their adult life, regardless of their basic constitutional type. Consequently, references to previously discussed remedies are essential for a thorough appreciation of *Nux vomica,* and in the following pages its personality picture will be liberally compared with, and differentiated from, those of other constitutional types—especially *Sulphur, Arsenicum,* and *Lycopodium.*

Nux, like *Sulphur,* is often employed as the opening remedy in cases in which a person must be cleansed of the ill-effects of previously used allopathic drugs. But it plays a more particular role in the individual who has been overdosed with herbal nostrums or homoeopathic medicines and who therefore cannot tolerate even the least "similar" medicine.* *Nux* stabilizes the oversensitive or over-reactive physique, so that a patient can again respond to his constitutional or a well-chosen remedy.

In its cleansing role, *Nux vomica* has also proved invaluable in cases of chemical sensitivities and severe reactions to toxins and pollutants in the environment. It further cleanses the constitutions of persons who in the relatively recent past have overindulged in recreational drugs, alcohol, tobacco, coffee, and other such stimulants (for substance or stimulant abuse in the more distant past, *Sulphur* is more efficacious). In cases of current substance addiction, *Nux* helps temper the craving, lessens the dependence, and eases the withdrawal symptoms. It is also often the preferred remedy for the digestive disturbances and ailments (including liver dysfunction) of those who are paying the price for their dietary indiscretions—notably overindulgence in foods that are too rich or highly seasoned. "My enjoyment of food has been woefully curtailed," one former appreciator of good wines and hot and spicy foods lamented; and another gourmet regretted his "asocial stomach" that prevented him from dining out and forced him to subsist on the blandest fare.

In his allergic reactions to the environment, however, *Nux vomica* most closely resembles *Arsenicum album*. With a nose like a bloodhound, he is sensitive to perfume, tobacco, different forms of vegetation, animal smells, dander, dust, and mold. He is also sensitive to bright light, which causes photophobia; to cold (conceivably, the hot and spicy food he craves, or alcohol, helps supply the warmth that he is always seeking); and is exceedingly alert to sounds. He can be driven distracted by sound above him or next door, even if it is just muffled voices or someone treading on the floor—and sleep, of course, is impossible; he is also unable to work if there is the slightest noise within earshot. Unlike *Sulphur,* who enjoys ambient noise and activity around him when he is working, or

---

*See the *Introduction* for further information.

Lycopodium, who also likes these when not too close (when they are taking place in the next room), *Nux* requires absolute quiet for concentration. Altogether, this oversensitive type displays a low tolerance for anything in the environment inimical to his nerves or his physique, including pain.

Just as he does physically, so *Nux* emotionally feels everything too strongly. Not only is he ardent in his likes and dislikes, but he also easily succumbs to fears and is beset by anxieties. Like *Arsenicum,* he may be inordinately concerned about the future, financial security, the physical safety of his family, or his own safety (one Wall Street broker admitted to always sitting in the middle car of his commuter train in case of a front-end or rear-end collision). But he does not worship as devotedly at the shrine of good health as does *Arsenicum,* giving the impression that visiting doctors is one of his foremost pleasures. Nor is he as susceptible to suggestion, feeling obligated to come down with every illness he reads about in the papers.

Moreover, he is not the frustrated would-be physician that *Arsenicum* so often appears to be; as a patient, he is content to be "the patient" and does not try to know more than the physician. If asked toward the end of the office consultation, "Have you told me all your symptoms?" the patient may reply, "I'm sure I haven't, but I'm equally sure you don't want to hear any more, so I will just stop here." (*Arsenicum* would be compelled to arrive at the end of the list.) In fact, more like *Lycopodium, Nux* may announce defiantly to the homoeopath in charge of his case, "You may as well know at the outset that you do not have my confidence and trust. So your medicines might not work on me." (The latter, of course, remains unperturbed. Just as the sun shines on the just and the unjust alike, so the homoeopathic remedies work equally well on believers and skeptics.)

It follows naturally that an individual who is so sensitive to disturbances in his physical environment, with nerves so easily frayed, will likewise be sensitive to any form of disharmony in his life.

Indeed, *Nux* is fastidiousness personified. Neatness, order, punctuality, and efficiency are as essential to him as to *Arsenicum,* and he exhibits the same perfectionism, the same attention to detail and delicate touch in whatever he sets out to do. Additionally, with his hypercritical nature it is equally difficult for him to be completely satisfied with his surroundings. A typical complaint is "My house/ office/back yard is a source of constant irritation. Wherever I look, something there is not right." His irritability is sparked when others disregard or disturb his own particular idea of order, and he likes things to be performed in a specific way ("the correct way"). Thus, he cannot enjoy half a grapefruit unless it is properly sectioned first, or he becomes upset at someone painting the garden fence with too small a brush ("Such an inefficient way of doing it!" he grumbles).

"Any job worth doing is worth doing *well,*" is his professed creed; and he ranks a mere notch below *Arsenicum*'s "Anything worth doing is worth overdoing." He might be able to tolerate (although barely) an unstraightened picture on the wall (which *Arsenicum* is unable to leave uncorrected) but cannot stand open drawers or gaping closet doors. The colleagues and students of one *Nux vomica* professor of English literature claimed they could find any book on his shelves blindfolded, so meticulously were they arranged by subject matter and century—and, of course, in alphabetical order. ("Everything in my office and in my home has its appointed place, and if someone moves it, I move it back.") Much of this striving for excellence, not to speak of the infinite care that he brings to all his undertakings, is admirable. But at times, the fastidiousness of *Nux,* like that of *Arsenicum,* becomes too much of a good thing—an obsession instead of a virtue. In this imperfect world, the individual is never at peace with himself and becomes a nuisance to others, who heartily wish for some liberating dirt, disorder, or inefficiency.

Nux vomica's hypersensitivity might further manifest as touchiness. He is quick to feel misunderstood and to escalate a misunderstanding into a grievance. If another fails to react in tune with his desires, he grows peevish ("No one ever listens to me! I am fast becoming a mere cipher in my own home!"). He is also quick to take offense and, prickly as a porcupine, bristles into instant defense ("Who's irritable? I'm not irritable. *You're* irritable," he snaps). When he is on edge, a piece of undercooked or overcooked meat served at home or in a restaurant is taken as a personal affront, and he may cause a scene. *Nux,* in fact, is expert at causing scenes, both in public and private; his fiery temper is notorious. Even when this aspect of his nature is controlled, he can be tight, testy, of uncertain mood. Every day his colleagues at work wonder what mood he will be in, and his wife asks herself the same question when he is on his way home, so as to adjust her behavior accordingly. Whether happy or discontented, prickly or benign, his mood must always be taken into consideration by those around him, and he may require constant humoring and placating. Yet all the while he himself complains of being harassed and talks of longing for tranquillity and repose.

Impatience is another pronounced feature of the personality picture. *Nux vomica* is always in a hurry, always feels pressed for time, and is bewailing its scarcity. He can be unduly impatient with himself if things don't go right the first time. The child stamps his foot and screams when he cannot achieve some result at once. The adult angrily throws down his work or wrestles irascibly with the physical obstacle that deters him in his task. And because he requires complete quiet to concentrate well, he becomes disproportionately impatient at interruptions when working ("Get out and leave me alone!"). He is also impatient at outside delays to his plans and desires, feeling that he must do something *at once* and force things his own way, instead of allowing events to take their natural course. He is impatient when requiring assistance; he wants it immediately—or would rather go without. To him, help delayed is help denied. Certainly, he grows impatient at others' slowness to learn or to understand and, like *Arsenicum,* is fault-finding with those who are less competent than himself. Also similar to *Arsenicum,* in his impatience to get things done, he drives others as hard as he does himself.

Another key word to the personality type is "spasmodic." In strychnine poisoning the most marked feature is spasms and convulsions, and the *Nux* physical picture includes various twitchings, tremblings, quiverings, and spasms—either of the entire body or of single parts (such as the colon, a limb, the spine), spasms of coughing or sneezing, spasmodic labor pains in the woman, and so on. On the emotional level, there are correspondingly short-lived but unbridled outbursts of irritability or ill-humor and a tendency to fly off the handle when provoked.

Such spasticity is exemplified in the *Nux* motorist: cars, driving, and trips bring out all that is aggressive, belligerent, and sarcastic in an otherwise perfectly pleasant individual. The type is notorious for fretting in traffic, fuming at a car cutting in ahead of him (while cutting into the faster lanes himself), and abusing other drivers. He is incensed at the suggestion that he may have taken a wrong turn, while being lost is the ultimate humiliation. *Nux vomica* is the dominant note in the tense, irritable father of the family in Ring Lardner's short story "The Young Immigrunts," who travel by automobile across the Midwest (written from the viewpoint of the young child):

> Heavens said my mother Ypsilanti must be a abnormal school to have such a large football field.
>
> My father wore a queer look. This is not Ypsilanti this is Ann Arbor he cried.
>
> But I thought you said we would go south of Ann Arbor and direct to Ypsilanti said my mother with a smirk.
>
> I did say that but I thought I would surprise you by coming into Ann Arbor replied my father . . . with a gastly smile.
>
> Personally I think the surprise was unanimous. . . .
>
> Well you would better stick to the main roads said my mother tacklessly.
>
> Well you would better stick to your own business replied my father with a pungent glance. . . .
>
> Are you lost daddy I arsked tenderly.
>
> Shut up he explained. . . .

Characteristic in this literary example is *Nux*'s refusal at times to even attempt to curb his temper. The shrewd and successful professional or business man can so completely forget himself in a petty outburst that, heedless or unaware of the impression he is making on others, he defies all civilized rules of behavior. The employer who cannot engage in a conversation without shouting, or talk on the telephone without slamming down the receiver in irritation before the other has finished his reply, and who reacts to every situation with intemperateness and excess may well require *Nux vomica.* Yet, only minutes after an exhibition of temper, he acts as if nothing untoward had happened. "I don't get ulcers, I *give* them," was one such person's pithy self-assessment. But ultimately *Nux* might develop ulcers himself. He is not as robust as *Sulphur,* who does truly forget his explosions and leaves his vexations behind. *Nux* may act as though he has forgotten, but he continues to sense the disharmony in the atmosphere, and this eats away at him.

A *Nux* banker sought homoeopathic aid for his ulcer pain. When asked about his memory and powers of concentration, he replied, "No problem there. It's my disposition that needs repairing, not my mind. I am blessed with the longest memory but the shortest temper known to man. In fact, people tell me I'm *the* most disagreeable person they've ever dealt with. Personally, I would settle for being just the *second* most disagreeable one. I might find life easier."

The remedy has repeatedly assisted in tempering those hair-trigger reactions, to permit a few seconds to elapse first. Then the individual may cool down sufficiently for reflection and, realizing that restraint is sometimes better than what he views as a fearless outspokenness, opt for a more measured response.

The *Nux vomica* woman is, on the whole, less hot-tempered than the man—less easily stirred to irascibility, quarrelsomeness, or loss of composure. But the hypersensitivity is there—the same overexcitation, overstimulation, and overreaction to the environment. And, certainly an unstable mood, a nervous irritability, a running criticism of others' shortcomings reminiscent of *Arsenicum album,* or a martyred querulousness reminiscent of *Sepia* ("Nobody realizes how much I suffer. But because I don't complain, I get no sympathy from anyone. . . .") are weaknesses the female *Nux vomica* will either contend with or indulge.

Since every constitutional remedy has its twofold aspects, *Nux vomica* may present the diametric opposite of the traditional picture of enervation, intemperance, or agitated anxiety. Although obviously high-strung, he is, like *Lycopodium,* outwardly calm, collected, and understated in manner—and moreover, acts as though unaware of his attractive qualities. Significantly, this self-contained person often emerges from a highly intense, vocal, and excitable family; but *he* has decided to be different. He will not raise his voice, betray his displeasure, or allow himself to harbor strong feelings about minor matters; at all times he will remain in command of his emotions. Further, because *Nux*'s emotions are close to the surface and his sensibilities acute, when he is on even keel he has more natural "sweetness" than the average male (a strange word to apply to *Nux vomica,* but appropriate). He can be intensely sympathetic, even weeping at affecting incidents with a *Pulsatilla*-like sentimentality, and be visibly affected by suffering in others. This is one of the few types that feels faint or can actually faint from the sight of blood. Additionally, suffering easily as he does from a tender pride, he is particularly careful not to pass on humiliation to another.

Another distinctive feature of the even-keeled type is a desire for self-improvement. He will deliberately and conscientiously apply himself to being tolerant and to curbing any self-serving proclivities in his dealings with people. A *Nux vomica* businessman at one point in his life arrived at the understanding that man, in being entrusted with the stewardship of this world, is responsible for protecting *all* vulnerable forms of life. Sparing no expense, he began restructuring and reorganizing his particular industry so as to be considerate of the environment, eliminate the use of animals in the testing and manufacturing of his products, and whenever possible, hire handicapped and disabled persons. To these ends he untiringly bent his efforts. Indeed, it is his steadfast efforts at self-improvement that gives to certain *Nux vomica* individuals a rare moral scrupulousness. Two centuries ago Hahnemann observed of the type, "clear consciousness of his existence; delicate, strong, proper feeling of right and wrong."

Sometimes the nature is blended: irascibility or an abrupt and testy manner alternating with sweetness, consideration, and true kindness. Regardless of how curt his manner and caustic his remarks, how unbridled his temper, under *Nux*'s abrasive exterior there often lies a soft heart and an undemonstrative rectitude. (The *Nux vomica* juxtaposition of virtues and defects differs, however, from that of the dualistic *Lachesis* in that he is more accepting of his own blended nature or less aware of it—consequently less at war with himself and projecting a less conflicted image.) Certainly, the wife and family of a *Nux* individual will often claim to sense a genuine concern and affection, and this consciousness offsets much that is rough or jagged on the surface. The wife of a *Lycopodium,* we recall, while seemingly having little to complain of her husband's impeccable behavior in public, may lament of some intangible deficiency, an impenetrable aloofness, in private. The reason may simply be that *Lycopodium* has less ardor, less emotional support to give, than the more fervent *Nux vomica.* Furthermore, in a happy family situation the attached *Nux vomica* husband might speak of his wife with generosity, volunteering touchingly and somewhat sentimentally, "She does not know how much she means to me, and how much she helps me! I simply cannot imagine life without her!" or "I consider every moment lost when I am not in her presence." *Sulphur, Lycopodium,* and *Arsenicum* would seldom express themselves in this manner, even if possessing similar feelings.

Conceivably, then, it is precisely *Nux vomica*'s heightened responsiveness, his more excitable nature that causes his romantic passions to run amok when he is thwarted or suffering from disillusionment. An excellent (if somewhat romanticized) literary portrait of the blended *Nux vomica* love nature is seen in Rhett Butler, the hero of *Gone With the Wind.* The disappointment of his true and ardent feelings for Scarlett O'Hara intensifies his inherent cynicism, harshness, and alcoholism—while he simultaneously exhibits an unexpected gentleness and understanding in his dealings with children and a sensitive, delicate appreciation of the fine qualities of Melanie Wilkes.

However, the classic picture of *Nux vomica* is not that of the romantic lover, but of the tense, driving, highly competitive, overstressed businessman or professional, caught up in the fast pace of modern life. He has been described as the overwrought, overworked town or city dweller who sits at his desk for long hours, sometimes late into the night—who receives many letters, many phone calls, and has a great many irons in the fire. All this forces him to hurry from one important matter to another; and when he finally does get home, his mind is too wound up to switch off, and he continues to think and worry about his work. The fretting prevents him from falling asleep and even if he does sleep, he does so fitfully and awakens unrefreshed—and querulous. Regarding eight uninterrupted hours of sleep as an inalienable human right, he complains of gross cosmic injustice when deprived of them ("I thought all God's creatures could at least sleep!").

Highly career-oriented and, like *Arsenicum,* commanding a strong work ethic, he welcomes new challenges and tends to deal with the stresses or anxieties of daily life by taking on *more* work. As intense in this sphere as he is in others, he finds it difficult setting limits here—especially as a sense of professional purpose is essential to his self-esteem. He is convinced that through work he proves his worth to the outside world. The self-made man who has toiled hard for what he has achieved and expects the same commitment from others—but who, at the same time, is convinced (often not without reason) that he can do things better himself and who therefore finds it difficult to delegate responsibility and insists on keeping a finger in every pie—is often *Nux vomica.*

The type is rightly considered clever. He is resourceful, mentally adroit, capable of change, and, by virtue of being the possessor of an orderly, methodical mind, whatever he promotes or sets out to accomplish is carried through systematically. Assuming that most problems can be resolved by effort and application and that hard work leads to success, he is painstaking first and confident afterward. Thus, he succeeds where another only talks of succeeding. And because he thinks fast under pressure, *Nux vomica* is highly represented among businessmen, journalists, surgeons, and court-room lawyers. Moreover, even when an artist or scholar he displays a practical turn of mind and a pragmatic approach to ideas. Unlike the *Sulphur* dreamer or idealist who becomes lost in abstractions or empty theorizing, *Nux* sees situations clearly and judges them realistically. His logical mind is capable of abstracting lessons from past experience and applying them to the future (a faculty that is not at all that common).

Being highly receptive to ideas and absorbing them easily, *Nux* might aspire to be a Renaissance man—well-rounded, multifaceted in his interests and talents, displaying pride of intellect, and believing in an aristocracy of culture. Goethe, "the last Renaissance man," as he has been called, is representative of the type. In contrast to the predominantly *Sulphur* mentalities of his distinguished compatriots, Kant, Marx, and Hegel, whose output can be traced back to a single all-embracing vision, the multifaceted Goethe engaged in many different disciplines—poetry, dramaturgy, novel writing, physiology, botany, economics, and politics—approaching each discipline on its own terms and with a thorough professionalism. Yet, even when striving to broaden his knowledge, *Nux vomica* remains highly discriminating. In his sensitivity to beauty (a form of the harmony and order he prizes highly) he responds to the minutiae of nature and art as well as to the grandeurs. He can be as profoundly stirred by the poise or tint of a wayside flower or the carved foliation on a piece of furniture as by the sweeping, all-inclusive grandeur of a *Sulphur* philosophical system.

He is sensitive to language and manipulates it well. Well-spoken himself, every chord of his being responds to a felicitous expression. If a foreigner, he at once picks up an interesting turn of phrase and uses it at the first opportunity; and the native is equally alert to new ways of expressing himself in his own language. His intellectual and verbal agility often make him a good conversationalist: sharp, pithy, quick at repartee—seldom boring. He is able to make his point concisely and does not, like *Sulphur,* deliver monologues or talk *at* people. Rather, he seeks a verbal give and take and tries to elicit a response from his interlocutor so as to continue a lively discussion. If he has a particular conversational weakness, it is to be acerbic, sarcastic, sharp-tongued.

An examination of power relationships is central to any analysis of *Nux vomica*. First of all, he is able to assert his authoritarian nature because of his indisputable competence, which propels him into positions of power and leadership, whatever his field. Thus positioned, he can then openly exercise his mighty organizational and strategic skills. But he is equally skilled at subtle and indirect manipulation of power relationships. He employs such tactics as attacking in pretended (or imagined) self-defense and is adept at guerrilla warfare—engaging in forays in the opponent's territory, then scurrying back to safety to await the next opportune occasion. *Sulphur* is also a good strategist and overall organizer but at times has difficulty attending to the practical details and is thus weaker in systematic implementation of his vision. The *Nux* mentality, excelling both in strategy and in the minutiae of tactical maneuvers, resembles *Arsenicum album* more.

Therefore, it goes almost without saying that *Nux vomica* enjoys making decisions and assuming responsibility on any level. His eyes light up with a special disciplinary gleam when he assumes control of a situation, leaving others little choice but to comply. Then, having once laid down the law, he expects unquestioning obedience and does not, like some types (especially *Natrum muriaticum*), enjoy the endless negotiation of differences of opinion. One man, when taking his family out to dine in a restaurant, would insist on dictating their choice of dishes. "You shouldn't order sole," he would protest to his wife. "You know this restaurant has poor fish. Order the lamb instead!" Or to his son, "How can you order a hamburger with french fries *again?* You chose that last time—and anyway, I don't bring you to restaurants to eat anything as primitive as a hamburger with french fries." He would then proceed to order something else for them both.

Thus, although *Nux vomica*'s wife is not quite the indentured servant of the occasional *Sulphur* or *Arsenicum* spouse, who must, through work and obedience, earn the right to live in her own house, still her status is often merely that of trusted retainer. One woman stated that what irritated most in her marriage was her husband's way of consulting her about various domestic arrangements (whom to invite for dinner, whether the trees in the yard should be pruned, what armchair to buy for that space in the living room) only *after* the decision had been carried out. "I was taken in by this pretense of joint household decisions until I realized there was no use in my volunteering an opinion, since the question was purely rhetorical. The guest had already been invited, the tree pruned, the armchair selected, and he had no intention of backing down or changing his mind." (Of course, as with *Arsenicum,* the gender roles can be reversed.) Moreover, in his assertion of power, *Nux* can be unreasonable. Although disposed to argue and contradict, *he* is intolerant of contradiction.

However, *Nux* is also able, when necessary, to submit to higher authority. One person described himself as follows: "At work I am most cooperative. In fact, like a good soldier, I am stupid and obedient and do what I'm told. But at home I am a dictator." To be sure, it is sometimes hard for the type to maintain relationships of equality.

Nux vomica's ready assumption of power and responsibility is as clearly exhibited in his professional life as in his personal one. Before you know it, a *Nux* has taken over management of the firm and is making all the important decisions; and, once established, he proceeds to move from strength to strength. Certainly, he shares with *Sulphur* and *Arsenicum* a strong entrepreneurial mentality. However, there is always the danger that power and success will go to his head and that he might undermine that which he has so relentlessly striven for and so assiduously built up. In fact, handling success is often a greater challenge to *Nux* than achieving it.

For all the reasons just mentioned and also because he is emblematic of the "blended" nature, no lesser a figure than Napoleon

Bonaparte will be examined as representative of the capable, authoritarian *Nux vomica* personality. Indeed, the intensity of Napoleon's nature, its greatness and glaring weaknesses, present the type's virtues and defects in sharp relief.

First and foremost, Napoleon epitomizes the highly practical and pragmatic *Nux* mentality ("God is on the side of the strongest battalions") that readily translates concepts into action. He possessed the ability to size up a situation realistically, to recognize the measures that had to be taken, and to take them at the opportune time ("The same thing cannot be done twice in the same century"). Moreover, his discarding of old-fashioned methods of warfare, with their cumbersome battle plans, and his introduction of the new factor of speed (*"Activité! Vitesse!"* ["Activity! Speed!"] he would repeat to his generals) are in keeping with the accelerated *Nux vomica* pace. Through *tempo* he was able to emerge victorious against overwhelming numerical odds, and this tempo was not confined to the battlefield. He imparted to the whole of Europe a speeding-up of social processes through which society was fundamentally transformed. It was Napoleon who ushered in the fast pace of modern life with which *Nux vomica* is so closely identified.

Further, Napoleon was extraordinary both for the Renaissance scope of his achievements (a strong intellect and lively curiosity helped him to become knowledgeable in history, geology, mathematics, and law) and for his *Nux vomica* ability to implement his vision and ideas once he had attained a foothold. The mere enumeration of his positive contributions suggests the range of his talents. He brought France out of post-Revolutionary chaos with amazing swiftness, ushering in a stage of prosperity through his social, economic, political, and religious reforms. He granted freedom of religion and of trade and extended judicial rights and civil security to all citizens and adopted measures to ease the economic pressures on the poor—for whom he harbored genuine sympathy (having come from a relatively poor background and being entirely a self-made man). He performed a signal service for administration by centralizing the government and giving it a form that has lasted to the present day.

The *Code Napoléon,* developed by lawyers and scholars working under his general guidance, remains the fundamental law of France.

His Renaissance-man attributes also encompassed a profound (if somewhat cynical) understanding of human nature and psychology. He thoroughly understood his fellow-countrymen and demonstrated an unerring instinct for what the masses wanted. He even accurately assessed his own *Nux* mentality when he said, "My greatest talent consists in my clear insight into everything . . . . Different affairs are all grouped in my head as in a desk. When I want to break off with one, I close its drawer and open another one. They never get mixed up. They don't confuse or tire me by their manifoldness." (However, the grandeur of his ideas, the breadth of his vision, and his capacity to forge the destinies of others suggest that some part of him was also *Sulphur.*)

But Napoleon also displayed *Nux vomica*'s weaknesses to an exaggerated degree. Vanity, power-hunger, and intoxication from success were the causes of his downfall. ("Three more years and I am master of the universe," he said in early 1812—three years before the Battle of Waterloo.) He had himself crowned Emperor of France despite his basically democratic and republican convictions; and, heedless of contrary advice, he pressed on with one war after another when France and the whole of Europe were crying out for peace.

Even Napoleon's physique, manner, and physical symptoms correspond to the *Nux* constitutional picture—the swarthy complexion, sharply chiseled features, and the nervous, masterful, irritable, impatient demeanor. (His reply to a subordinate general requesting a favor is typical: "Ask of me anything you want, sir, except time!") And his very ailments were true to type. His defeat at the Battle of Waterloo has been attributed partially to a severe attack of *Nux*-like hemorrhoids (worse from the least movement, better sitting), which forced him to remain seated in his tent during crucial stretches of the four-day battle in lieu of commanding his troops in the field. Unable to observe the fighting first-hand, he made uncharacteristic mistakes.

Thus, *Nux vomica* will often start out in life as a responsive and high-minded individual, but one not overly supplied with equanimity. He exhibits force, but it is an uncertain force, and life's harsh lessons, disappointments, or a disharmonious environment can bring out the irascible, intemperate, quarrelsome side of his disposition. The more fortunate *Nux* individual, however, whose sensitivities have not been unduly challenged, who has not been overly subjected to hardship and emotional stress (including too rapid a rise to success), or who has consciously applied himself to cultivating temperance, tolerance, and composure will display a graciousness and probity which, when combined with the type's native cleverness and strong feelings, make for a truly interesting and fine personality.

Nux vomica

PRINCIPAL REGIONS AFFECTED

Head   Headache in occiput and over eyes; **vertigo** with reeling (as if intoxicated); pain as if a nail were driven in— sometimes with light sensitivity; **migraine**, sometimes with **nausea and vomiting; head colds with stuffy nose and much sneezing**

Respiration   **Oversensitivity to the external environment** disposes the type to allergies, hayfever, asthma; head colds with much sneezing; chest colds with paroxysms of coughing and oppressed breathing

Digestion   **Various affections of the liver, gallbladder, and bowels** cause cramping, nausea, vomiting; retching, biliousness, feelings of weight in stomach, or pressure as from a stone for several hours after eating; heartburn; **constipation, with ineffectual urging or incomplete and unsatisfactory movement**; diarrhea; hemorrhoids

Urinary   Irritable bladder; frequent calls with ineffectual or incomplete urge

Male   High sexual energy; **easily excited desire**; complaints from sexual excesses, including impotence

Female   Weepy before menses; migraine headaches before or during menses; severe cramping with pain in sacral area; nausea and vomiting or constant desire to stool; excessive bleeding at menopause; inefficient or ineffectual labor pains

Back   **Affections of the spine** (anywhere along the cerebrospinal axis); spasms, cramping; muscle tension; must sit up to turn in bed

Nerves   **Easily irritated: heightened sensitivity to noise, odors, light; intolerance of pain; sleeplessness from anxious thoughts of day's problems,** rush of ideas; wakens around 3:00 to 4:00 AM, starts thinking about work, and cannot get back to sleep again until morning; then wakens grumpy and unrefreshed; dreams are anxious, full of hurry, confusion, or of disturbing events of previous day

GENERALITIES

A key symptom is the incomplete, unsatisfactory feeling that accompanies the ineffectual urging to expel: bowels, urine, expectoration, undigested food (wants to but cannot vomit); the infant (in labor), etc.

Continued.

Nux vomica—cont'd

GENERALITIES—cont'd

Violent nature of many ailments; spasmodic complaints, with twitching, trembling

High physical and mental energy (nervous), which the individual tends to overtax by overworking or unhealthy living

Ill-effects of alcohol, coffee, or other stimulants, recreational drugs, allopathic, or other forms of medication

MODALITIES (< worse; > better)

Time < Early morning; 4:00 PM; monthly

> Evening (night energy)

Temperature < Cold: open air, draft, wind, uncovering

> Warmth in every form: sun, clothing, food and drink

Position < Sitting

> Being active; lying on something hard (in affections of the spine); lying down when resting

Food/Drink < Rich, hot spicy foods (which he craves); alcohol, coffee, or other stimulants (which he craves)

> Warm drinks (such as milk); fats (which he tolerates well)

Other < Retention (despite urging) of whatever the body is trying to expel

> Expelling whatever the body is retaining

GUIDING MENTAL SYMPTOMS

Especially suited to the adult male rising in his profession who is overstressed—and as a result, is tense, irritable, and short-tempered

Ambitious, hard-working, competitive, and commanding personality—but success might go to his head

Strong intellect, but fault-finding; also self-critical; intolerant of contradiction and of poor performance in others; impatient

Competent, clear-thinking, well organized, but at times overly fastidious; too easily frustrated by small things

Emotional sensitivity: complaints from anger, excitement, strong feelings

Unstable temper with poor self-control—easily upset and offended; or, conversely, exceptionally controlled and mentally refined

Fears illness, impending accidents; poverty

Natrum muriaticum

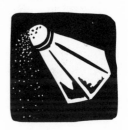

Ye are the salt of the earth.
—*Matthew* 5:13

atrum muriaticum is sodium chloride or common table salt, an everyday substance with a number of unique properties. Salt absorbs, retains, and condenses; it also crystallizes and preserves; and salt brings out the taste of other foods. These properties are clearly manifested in this personality type.

From youth onward, impressions are deeply absorbed and tenaciously retained by the *Natrum muriaticum* individual. On the positive side, this makes for a compassionate individual who is sensitive to others' wants and longings, loyal in affections, and appreciative of kindness. All too often, however, he is prone to absorb and retain unhappy impressions and then allows them to fester. He too vividly remembers past sorrows and hangs on to resentments. Where another would long ago have dismissed an unpleasant experience or irretrievable loss and gone on to other things, the inconsolable *Natrum muriaticum* remains stuck and cannot recover. To him, time is not the Great Healer. On the contrary, it serves only to solidify, then crystallize, the painful past, which then becomes magnified and holds him captive. Like a miser who hoards his gold and periodically goes to the strongbox to count it, *Natrum muriaticum* hoards his memories of injury and loss, periodically retrieving them for re-examination.

Frequently, the source of the problem is family. More than any other constitutional type, *Natrum muriaticum* suffers from a poor relationship with one or both parents. Part of his difficulty lies in his own inability to communicate to them his need for approval or support. By nature introverted, he is neither demonstrably affectionate nor an easy child to raise, but still he wants to be understood without having to explain himself. And the scars he bears from past parental inability to meet his emotional needs ("They never even *tried* to understand me!"), not to speak of their unwanted advice or explicit or implied disapproval, can breed a lifetime of retained grievances. It was a *Natrum muriaticum* who explained in all seriousness that he lost faith in his parents and consequently in humanity, when, as a child of seven, he discovered there was no Santa Claus. "My parents *lied* to me," he exclaimed indignantly. "So how could I ever trust them or anyone else again?" It takes but that little to reawaken all the disappointments of childhood and the attendant resentments.

In his insistence on complete understanding, the type could be viewed as making excessive demands. Yet, paradoxically, often it is *Natrum muriaticum* who, for all his hang-ups and feelings of being imposed on, is the child that harbors most devotion to his parents and is most likely to live with or next door to them so as to care for them in their old age. Further, his relations with his own children are generally good; having himself suffered so severely from the parental relationship, he is determined to be extra sensitive to their needs.

If he finds no excuse for injury in the parental relationship, *Natrum muriaticum* may seize on some other relationship formed relatively early in life at which to take offense: it might have been with a friend, teacher, sibling, or some family member whom he views as refusing to do his share. He does not necessarily display his grudge at the time of injury, but elephant that he is, he never forgets—and subsequently projects his unhappy experience onto the world at large. Indeed, something in his very nature leads one to suspect the type of seeking injury; or, to word it more accurately, of placing himself in situations in which injury is likely to occur.

However, it is essential to bear in mind that a salt diathesis develops not only when an individual is unable to overcome routine, everyday disappointments—not only when he needlessly cultivates painful memories and dwells on the past (so that like Lot's wife in the Bible, he is turned into a pillar of salt for looking back), but also in consequence of legitimate emotional traumas: the loss of a loved one through death or desertion, a painful humiliation or betrayal, an abusive parent or spouse, a bitter divorce, or disappointing children. The salt picture likewise emerges in those unfortunates who are trapped in difficult, no-way-out marriages or are enduring near-insoluble family situations, as well as in those dutiful persons who must bear the burden of others' selfishness or irresponsibilities. Finally, it emerges in those who find themselves in the ungratifying, guilt-ridden position of fearing they are not doing enough for another while still doing far more than they want—and more than anyone else.

Frequently, this type projects an aura of heaviness: there is heaviness in the lines around the eyes and in those running down from his nose to the corners of the mouth, and in his hangdog expression. He might display the habit of resting his head on his hand, as if to help the neck support it, or he walks with a heavy tread, with shoulders bowed, as if from carrying the weight of the world on them. These characteristics could be regarded as outer manifestations of a burdened nature—of one who is forever questioning, "Why is man subject to so much suffering, injustice, and loneliness?" It is *Natrum muriaticum* who in his very person suggests the unalterably tragic makeup of this world. At the same time, he is profoundly convinced that he has some important lesson to learn from these burdens and consequently is good at stoically enduring hardship.

Even while others would acknowledge the legitimacy of his injuries and grievances, *Natrum muriaticum* often becomes his own worst enemy in his passage through life by allowing the sorrowful aspects of human existence to be the lens through which he views reality. An apposite term for his distorting lens is *bleakness,* implying as it does an ultra-attunement to the minor-key forces at work in the world. Following are a few examples of *Natrum muriaticum*'s "bleak" physical or emotional response to the conventional symbols of life, beauty, joy.

Cheering, colorful, lovely spring, the season of regeneration and rebirth, is not only a time of physical aggravation but is also felt by him to be deceptive—its short-lived brightness serving only to remind man of the transience of beauty, the brevity of life, and the dissolving forces of nature. Even more, the bright warming sun, representing as it does the supreme stimulus of growth and life on earth, is poorly tolerated by him. Because he feels either enervated or drained by its direct rays, or is prone to headaches, he associates it with burning, fatigue, pain, and depletion. And since salt absorbs and retains water, humidity affects him adversely as it does few other types. On the other hand, the bracing, cool freshness of morning also finds him feeling tired, dejected, reluctant to rise and face another burdensome day ("How will I survive it?"). Conversely, his spirits lift in the evening, once the sun has set and he can sigh a relieved, "Whew! I managed to live through this day! Now I can rest."

Many of the beauties of art and nature oppress him. Because of its capacity to evoke memories better left untapped, beautiful music saddens him. Majestic mountains surrounding him bring on claustrophobia, while their exhilarating heights might bring on the fear of some sudden, uncontrolled impulse to fling himself down. As for the ocean—the salt-permeated matrix of all life, with all its symbolic associations with the primordial past—it is bound to provoke a complex set of reactions and to aggravate him even as it draws him ("I don't know why I keep coming back to it. I never feel good by the sea, but for some reason I can't stay away"). This last characteristic, incidentally, exemplifies an important aspect of *Natrum muriaticum:* to be hurt by that which he loves best. A person who has a passion for flowers is allergic to their scent; another who loves animals finds himself growing increasingly sensitive to their fur or dander; yet another falls ill every time he plans to visit a place or person he longs to see; and so on.

Furthermore, it is difficult for *Natrum muriaticum,* whose nature is essentially serious, to experience fun. He seldom feels carefree and comfortable at social gatherings, parties, or family celebrations—in part because he finds it exceedingly difficult to deal with persons whose thinking is not entirely in tune with his and of whom he does not entirely approve. Holidays, especially the Christmas season, are the worst time of the year for him. When everyone is supposed to be full of the holiday spirit and many are truly enjoying themselves, he becomes dejected, morose, and more aware than ever of man's intrinsic loneliness. In general, happiness to him is ephemeral. How can anyone experience lasting happiness when loss awaits one just around the corner and suffering is encountered at every turn? Happiness is merely a temporary break from the true tenor of the world. Even a smile to him is, as one *Natrum muriaticum* put it, "but a brave effort to cover up tears." Yet he himself often displays the loveliest of smiles—one that literally transforms his face, as all traces of heaviness and dejection vanish.

Above all, there is romantic love! With its enormous potential for pain, disappointment, and sorrow, *Natrum muriaticum* is fated to be caught here at his most vulnerable. Much of the grief he brings on himself by seeking out the company of one in whose presence he suffers—like a hovering moth repeatedly burning itself on a candle, but unable to stay away. Likewise, this type simply cannot put a love that is over and finished behind him. ("You don't stop loving a person just because he's hurt you. You can't forget a person just because he's left you." Or, "I don't separate easily from anyone I've once loved." Or, "How can I stop loving her? She was a part of me—and will never cease being a part of me—even though she's no longer around.") Even if the love is requited, he may place himself in an insoluble situation, courting a relationship that will inevitably lead to grief. He falls in love with a married woman or fantasizes about someone so unsuitable as to be unattainable. This trait has been encapsulated in the image of the grand lady who falls in love with her coachman. To *Natrum muriaticum,* romantic love is a complex, tortured emotion—all too often the source of profound sadness, unappeasable longing, and lasting ill-health.

It is, in fact, his bleak outlook that contributes to *Natrum muriaticum*'s "aloneness"—that almost ineradicable sense of not belonging anywhere in the world. Even when participating in a pleasant group situation, he feels left out or ill at ease. In any gathering larger than a very few close, like-minded friends, he feels superfluous. Moreover, holding steadfast to the conviction that no one can assist him in his loner status, he will not allow himself the comfort of friends or family. More than any other type, *Natrum muriaticum* rejects consolation or any outside attempt to extricate him from his isolation. Thus, he will still clutch onto the quirks and hang-ups that distance him from others as if they were his sole source of security in an insecure world. One man claimed, "Neuroses are like a blanket; they can be protective as well as terribly smothering. So when I seemed to be losing them, I felt not only lighter, but more exposed." *Natrum muriaticum* feels threatened at the very thought of having to relinquish his protective cloak or somehow to change (after all, salt *preserves*).

A Jungian analyst, Edward Whitmont, has advanced the thesis that this constitutional type represents man in search of his Ego. That is, he is in that period of his mental or spiritual development when he is breaking away from the "collective unconscious"—from family, heredity, traditional religious beliefs, class or cultural values—and is seeking to find his own true nature. But between the breaking from the past and attaining a higher integration (represented by discovery of the ego) there lies a transitional stage that is, of necessity, a lonely one. "Whenever the demands of the transition prove greater than the strength of the personality, a state of pathology ensues which has its remedy in *Natrum muriaticum*," writes Whitmont. "At the same time [he concludes], his state of isolation is accentuated by the fact that love, sympathy, and communion with others are longed for; yet an inner command forbids their acceptance and urges him to find the source of strength within himself."*

Natrum muriaticum, then, is the loner whose life is complicated by a need for companionship. Constantly vacillating between a desire both for the isolation he requires to resolve his deep inner problems and also for companionship to help him endure them, he is never completely satisfied either with people or without. Because he finds relationships fraught with potential pain and misunderstandings, he might attempt to eschew them. To avoid being emotionally injured, he tries to surround his heart with a thick wall ("A thick, impenetrable wall of scar tissue," said one woman of herself, who was determined never again to be placed in a position of being deeply humiliated or wounded). But although the loner talks of living far away from people in a beach shack or a cabin in the woods, if he does exile himself from society, he eventually grows tired of living in glorious isolation—and returns to where he can interrelate with people, even at the risk of emotional injury.

Curiously, *Natrum muriaticum,* who is subject to the most relentless sadness, is also distinguished by the intensity of his hopes and dreams, which alone offer him respite from his customary burdened, introspective self. It does not take much to spark them off and launch them into unrealistic realms. Dreams of ideal friendships, wild romances, or spectacular accomplishments can occupy him for years while he lives his humdrum existence; and sometimes they satisfy him as if they were reality. The socially concerned individual is full of idealistic longings. He has unlimited faith (not necessarily confirmed by experience) in man's capacity for self-improvement, and dreams that the fabric of society will change once humanity understands its own best interests—and good, honest, conscientious people are put to the task. When he waxes enthusiastic over some Utopian dream, his eyes light up, his complexion gains color, and

*Edward C. Whitmont, *Natrum muriaticum,* The Homoeopathic Recorder, Vol. LXIII, No. 5, November 1947, p. 121.

his whole person sparkles. Since the past is full of painful memories and the present is burdensome, only the future promises happiness and fulfillment.

The classic deterrent to melancholy, however, is laughter, and the heart of the most introverted *Natrum muriaticum* can best be reached, not by kindness or the display of affection, not by sympathy or consolation, but by laughter. He does not necessarily possess a better sense of humor than other types, but he more greatly appreciates another's humor. However profound his despondency, inconsolable his loss, unappeasable his grief, or impregnable his isolation, it cannot withstand the assault of humor. This alone disarms him, engendering self-forgetfulness, unblocking emotions, and opening a line of communication between his secluded self and the outside world.

Natrum muriaticum's response to humor runs the gamut of various types of laughter—from the uncontrollable schoolgirl giggle to explosive guffaws. In between lie the loud cackle, betraying an element of discomfort when some sensitive point has been dealt with humorously, as well as immoderate laughter, where he laughs too heartily for the occasion, and the bursts of spasmodic or involuntary laughter (which are, of course, a release of pent-up emotions—hence their uncontrolled nature). Then, too, there can be a strained quality to his cheerfulness, a false hilarity, or an underlying hysterical note. Or the type may emit a nervous little laugh at something not at all funny or give an inappropriate smile when he is narrating a serious or sad event. This last reflects not lack of feeling, but unease—an attempt to put on a good face, so as not to betray his despair.

As a rule, *Natrum muriaticum* manifests reticence and reserve. He experiences little pleasure in disclosing the deeper recesses of his soul—while keeping a stiff upper lip in the face of adversity is one of his strongest behavioral codes. True, occasionally he appears open and confiding, but the impression is deceptive. One learns his opinions about politics, religion, education—his tastes and preferences in art, sports, clothes, and food—but little about him personally. As to his inability to express emotions: sadness can rob him of the power of speech, and often he is too constricted inside to cry. Although tears may well up in his eyes from anger or frustration or when deeply moved by another's hardships, they do not *flow* easily—and he finds it especially difficult to cry when grieving for himself. When he does do so, it is alone in his room, in broken, choking sobs that catch painfully in the throat and bring on a headache. Just as his grief is too deep for consolation, so it is too fundamental, too all-pervasive for tears. Nevertheless (and this is idiosyncratic of the type), once the reticent individual does unbend and the long-repressed emotions finally surface, it is like a dam bursting. Then it all pours out—accompanied by a blotchy face and neck, bright red nose, and uncontrollable sobs. However, this flood of tears is not always healing; sometimes it resembles more a tropical rainstorm that leaves the atmosphere heavier than before. In pouring out his troubles, *Natrum muriaticum* works himself up into such a state that he aggravates his physical or mental condition.

He might also be tongue-tied when hearing of another's sorrow or may be prompted to make some inappropriate remark. This makes him appear distant or unfeeling, yet underneath he takes to heart what others tell him. Quick to sense the injuries and thwarted longings of others, every chord in him responds to their misery, and he may suffer more than they do. They eventually get over the loss or disappointment, but he continues to brood. Indeed, no constitutional type displays a greater capacity for vicarious suffering. When he has no personal or professional reason to suffer, he identifies with the injured or oppressed. ("Not only am I miserable, but something in me is *determined* to be miserable. If I find nothing to be miserable about in my own life, I will find it in someone else's!") This is the individual who, with so many emotional problems of his own to be resolved, still allows himself to become emotionally embroiled in matters that are really not his concern. One *Natrum muriaticum* will claim to be emotionally exhausted from trying to straighten out a sibling's marital troubles; another is depressed be-

cause a friend's son is imposing on his parents; a third is anxious because a thoughtless colleague is giving trouble to his employer. The
victims themselves do not (to his indignation) seem to be overly
troubled, but this just makes him more determined to set things
right. It is with *Natrum muriaticum* more than with any other personality type that one is tempted to cry out, "Let others resolve their
own problems. Take care of yourself first!"

For all his heaviness and propensity for courting misery, *Natrum muriaticum* is a likable personality. He has character, solid virtues, and an undeniable high-mindedness. He is prepared to stick
tenaciously to his ideals and when promoting some cause he genuinely promotes *it* rather than himself personally. He is a considerate and thoughtful friend, steady and reliable in times of stress and,
like Dr. Watson to another's Sherlock Holmes, is ever willing to relinquish the limelight and support another's strength. Moreover, the
type's faithfulness is a byword. Those long-suffering heroines in
eighteenth and nineteenth century novels who wait patiently and un-
complainingly throughout 400 pages of hardship, grief, and yearning
for the obtuse heroes *finally* to recognize their solid worth and grow
to love them (think of Agnes Wickfield in Charles Dickens' *David
Copperfield*), are indubitably *Natrum muriaticum.*
He is thus a good person, usually motivated by kindness. But
sometimes, as with salt, a little goes a long way—and too much *Natrum muriaticum* in the constitutional picture breeds its own set of
difficulties. For instance, he might doggedly assert his own peculiari-
ties, demanding universal acceptance of them. Or he is highly argumentative, proving that he is, always has been, and always will be
right. To admit to error or a change of opinion is a humiliation,
while to apologize is sheer agony ("I'd rather die than say I'm
sorry"). Thus, while insecure in his social behavior, he is not insecure in his opinions and understanding. He knows (or thinks he
knows) what's right and will fight desperately on every front to defend this rightness—seldom knowing when to stop or retire from an
unprofitable scene of conflict. One of his hardest life lessons is to

learn that he could accomplish so much more (and so much more easily) if he did not perceive compromise or flexibility to be a threat to his very identity. The unbudging *Natrum muriaticum* here reflects the solidifying nature of salt; frequently he must receive a number of hard knocks before his unbending pillar-of-salt personality or crystallized patterns of behavior can change.

Sometimes the type is wanting in natural elegance and ease. There is a certain awkwardness in his build, movements, and bearing, and he may be lacking in the social graces. All angles and abruptness, taciturn and loquacious in spurts, he wishes he were inconspicuous in society, and in his extreme self-consciousness, he suffers from the often groundless conviction that everyone is looking at and judging him. His unease is most readily betrayed by his unsteady eyes. The eyes have traditionally been regarded as the "windows" or "interpreters" of the soul, and *Natrum muriaticum* dislikes strangers peering into his soul and reading his true feelings. Therefore, except with close friends, he is unable to make or maintain eye contact. His glance will shift up, down, or ever so slightly to the side instead of looking another straight in the eye. Furthermore, just as he displays pleasure in the way his whole face lights up, so he cannot hide his displeasure. He may not say anything outright, but his face (to his infinite chagrin) is always easy to read. He can also be honest and outspoken to the point of tactlessness. But then, even when he tries to be tactful, he is a poor liar, and once again, his face invariably betrays him.

Finally, this is the person who excuses, justifies, and explains himself too much, thereby placing himself further in the wrong. He is aware of this weakness but cannot help himself—and years later, writhes in mortification at the recollection of some incident. For instance, a *Natrum muriaticum* department chairman invited a younger professor to teach a summer course. "We are really scraping the bottom of the barrel. Our best teachers don't want to remain in the city during the summer, so I thought of you—" Then, recollecting himself and with a look of dismay, he compounded his gaucherie by trying to right it: "Of course, you are not the scrapings—

what I meant was . . ." and continued in this fashion until his interlocutor felt like crying out, "Just drop it! Forget it! It's all right, I'm not offended."

Natrum muriaticum often possesses a prominent unconventional streak. He has difficulty adapting to established values or the prevailing mode, despite genuine efforts to acclimatize. Something in his very bones attracts him to the outsider, the minority, the underdog, and he refuses to be impressed by what is popularly accepted or praised. This unconventionality can be displayed in a lack of interest in material things; he is satisfied with enough worldly goods for his simple needs, and his clothes reflect this. The president of an old established Boston firm will wear a threadbare suit and neatly starched shirt with frayed collar and cuffs. A *Natrum muriaticum* woman is seldom stylish, preferring above all to be comfortable in an old dress ("as long as it fits, why stop wearing it?") and in her sturdy, practical, too obviously healthy-for-the-feet shoes. With so many world problems to resolve—saving the whales or baby seals, nuclear disarmament, promoting homoeopathy or some other worthy but unpopular cause—she has no time for superficialities.

Likewise, in the realm of food, duty as much as taste determines *Natrum muriaticum*'s choice. If he is convinced that vegetables and legumes are virtuously in tune with the universe, he will conscientiously set about eating these three times a day, all the while insisting he loves nothing better. Often, then, his diet, clothes, tastes, and behavior reflect a strong sense of principled and moral obligation to the world, as well as a streak of self-denial ("I find myself forcing myself to do what I most dislike or not doing that which I most wish to do"). All these characteristics reaffirm his innate conviction that life is a serious business and that man is placed here on earth for duty, hard work, and no mean share of suffering.

Generally speaking, *Natrum muriaticum*'s tastes tend to be one-sided. Just as he might eat the same food day after day for months on end, or wear the same clothes (as if seeking security in predictable apparel or a monotonous diet), so if asked what type of book he favors, he will admit to reading only fiction or only history or only biographies or only mysteries or only books relating to his particular field—and these days especially, only books on health and self-improvement. A more immoderate type might become enamored of one particular book and spend many months rereading it. By the same token, he may listen to some favorite piece of music or see the same movie innumerable times. He might try to diversify, acquiring knowledge outside his specific area of interest, but without success. He cannot honestly enjoy or even appreciate whatever he is not attuned to at the moment and returns with relief to his tried and true favorites, on whose emotional impact he can completely rely. Paralleling these one-sided tastes are his one-sided talents. Even the best *Natrum muriaticum* minds carve deep, narrow grooves for themselves and remain in them. This can encourage the type to be a Johnny-one-note—thinking and talking only of the one subject that grips him. On the positive side, however, a focused determination helps him to overcome all obstacles and contributes to his success.

Representative of this last trait is Abraham Lincoln, whose rise to the Presidency was the result of a determined and persevering deepening of his groove. Lincoln actually embodied a number of *Natrum muriaticum* characteristics. He lost his mother at an early age and never got over the bereavement. Although his stepmother was wonderfully supportive, the sadness that never really left him has traditionally been attributed to his mother's death. Gawky in appearance and angular in manner, Lincoln was also known for his love of a good joke and readiness to laugh. He seldom gave way to the chronic melancholy that was an essential part of his nature, but instead found relief in the humorous stories he was constantly reading and quoting. The scene of the beleaguered Lincoln sitting with a book in the Oval Office at the height of the Civil War and laughing out loud is well known. When asked how he could laugh when so many men were dying on the battleground, he replied, "If I didn't find this vent for my sorrow, I would perish." The reserved Lincoln did not say such things lightly. Ironically, the author of the Gettys-

burg Address then added that he would gladly trade all he had accomplished in life to write like the (now long forgotten) minor humorist he was reading. Above all, his personality—solitary ("the
lonely man in the White House") and burdened with grief—somehow made it all the more appropriate that his *Natrum muriaticum*
shoulders should carry the tragedy of the Civil War.

Natrum muriaticum might also possess a one-sided or eccentric
memory. While he may forget in which century the Thirty-Year War
occurred after just having read a book on the subject, his memory
for what people say can be exceptional. He will recall whole sec-
tions of conversations heard in the past. If a person contradicts what
he said twenty years earlier, *Natrum muriaticum* feels disoriented—
even indignant: "You said before . . . Now you're telling me . . . What
exactly is it that you think?" That the person might be in a different
mood or view the situation from a different angle is highly disturbing to one who sets an inordinate store by consistency.

Although no one values consistency and predictability more
than a *Natrum muriaticum,* he himself is prone to sudden and
strange reversals. As a rule he is ultrareliable, possessing a bulldog-
like tenacity that compels him to hang on to a given situation, relationship, or chosen path at all costs; also, his fixed nature makes it
hard for him to shift gears. Unshakeably loyal and always dutiful, he
is prepared to make sacrifices for the sake of whatever cause or cru-
sade he espouses. But despite his outward solidity, his underlying
emotional state can be surprisingly unstable. Like a candle that
abruptly goes out for want of anything left to burn, seemingly over-
night he becomes indifferent to an ardent conviction or to an attach-
ment of many years' standing. A man or woman will one day, without warning, walk out on what appeared to be a perfectly happy
marriage—only throwing out in explanation, "It seemed the right
thing to do." Alternately, *Natrum muriaticum* decides to marry
someone he has known for years as a friend but has never considered marrying until that moment. Thus the type makes the most important decisions purely, as it seems, on impulse. But the reality is

that some growing inner intuition suddenly crystallizes into an un-shakeable resolution—and for the unbending individual, the break, or the decision, is final. So irrevocable is it, in fact, that he can hardly remember when he felt differently. It is as if, fearing lest he share the fate of Lot's wife for looking back, he takes it upon himself to *obliterate* the past.

Another facet of the *Natrum muriaticum* unpredictability is encountered in the unexpected rages, instigated by a dispute over a relatively minor issue, to which this normally self-restrained individual may be subject. With him it is not the heavy burdens but the straw that breaks the camel's back. To an outsider, his response might appear to be an irrational overreaction, suggestive of imbalance. But such behavior fits his pattern of enduring inequities, hardship, or abuse until he cannot bear the situation a minute longer—and the inevitable explosion occurs. Thus, there is method in *Natrum muriaticum*'s sudden impulsive anger, even as there is some madness in his method. The madness lies in his refusal to take constructive steps earlier in the proceedings, while he is still calm. To avoid unpleasantness, he chooses not to confront the offender, but to allow resentment to build up. Then some trifle sets him off and he reacts in an extreme fashion, incomprehensible to others.

In other words, although his behavior might be morally justified, politically it is not. The misunderstandings and deterioration of important relationships are partly the fault of his inability to be straightforward with people and state his needs. This pattern is especially apparent in family situations. A *Natrum muriaticum* woman might do more than her share in caring for her elderly parents and will lament to a friend that other family members are not pulling their weight. The obvious reaction of the friend is to ask, "Have you talked it over with them and divided the responsibility in a way that is satisfactory to all of you?" It then materializes that she has not done so because "It wouldn't work. No one will stick to the agreement."

"Well, why don't you just try. Confront them and say in so many words that you are feeling imposed on."

"What's the use? If after all these years they don't see the inequity for themselves, they will never understand."

"Still, you should try."

"I'm hoping they will understand without my having to tell them. They *should* realize that I'm doing all the work . . ."—thereby trying to make the mountain come to her, rather than taking a few steps into the foothills herself.

Even though underlying *Natrum muriaticum*'s inability to express his displeasure is a sincere reluctance to impose on or hurt others, he also dreads being offended by their wounding remarks in return. The type is extremely sensitive to unpleasantness directed at him. This aversion induces him to take a convoluted approach; his feelings are clear-cut, but his manner is evasive. In an attempt to act nobly or to endure, and especially to avoid confrontation, he is not straightforward. Then, to his astonishment, even indignation, others are irritated—and the resultant rupture is the more severe.

Shakespeare's play *King Lear,* one of the most concentrated fictional treatises on the nature of the salt diathesis ever penned, illustrates how convoluted relations can lead to desperate misunderstandings. The characters wander about on the heath, physically so close to each other and yet emotionally so distant—so unable to communicate and to unravel their differences—that all their true and honorable feelings go to waste. Not only is Lear himself a true *Natrum muriaticum* in seizing on an imagined insult, exaggerating it beyond reason and reaching the thoroughly erroneous conclusion that his daughter, Cordelia, has betrayed him—then undergoing circuitous and wrongheaded rationalizations to deny his love for her; Cordelia herself is constitutionally almost pure salt in her emotional self-consciousness, inability to express filial love in the correct words and gestures, as well as in her inflexible honesty and intransigent refusal to humor her old father's whims. Ironically, it is her uncompromising integrity that brings on the tragic events of the play. Even the noble and devoted Edgar is *Natrum muriaticum* in his (partly self-imposed) martyrdom, silently enduring his father's injustices as he cares for him in his blindness; also the loyal retainer, Kent, who, though banished by Lear, remains faithfully at his side in disguise, attempting (unsuccessfully, of course) to protect him from further folly. Each character must play out his role alone, unable to be helped or to help others, and each one must learn the hard way. Misunderstanding thus prevails to the end, when it is too late for mending.

While he might have difficulty relating socially or with family, *Natrum muriaticum* readily adopts the role of teacher, missionary, social worker, counselor, or helper with the handicapped or under-privileged. The truth is, he is often most at ease with those less fortunate or less enlightened than himself. Even if the work is emotionally draining, he will staunchly persevere if he thinks it will establish better communication among individuals and help them avoid the suffering to which he himself has been subjected. Helping others is an almost religious imperative with him. In counseling (in which role he has no superior) he is confident and positive, with none of his personal melancholy or insecurity showing through. Although he is convinced that he can teach others how best to live, he evinces no personal arrogance—conveying more of a "Do as I say" manner than *Lycopodium*'s "Be as I am." Like the proverbial unmarried marriage counselor, he is able to help others attain a health and happiness that he himself may never experience. It is *Natrum muriaticum* above all other personality types whose benevolence is a substitute for the love that is lacking in his own life and who, when he finds insufficient personal fulfillment in life, takes to good works on a large scale, helping the downtrodden, the oppressed, and those in pain.

In this way the type resembles the substance from which the remedy originates; he is indeed the "salt of the earth." Just as salt enhances the taste of food, so others' lives are enhanced by his ever-supportive role. But the relationship is symbiotic. Without food, salt cannot display its enhancing qualities, and without people to counsel and assist (thus diluting his concentrated salt properties), *Natrum muriaticum* dries up and withers emotionally—proving the truth of the saying "Too much salt makes a man dry." His performance of good works thus carries a self-serving aspect: he needs to be needed. Not only does he take satisfaction in guiding others, but in so doing he also is hoping to climb out of the Slough of his own Despond ("Perhaps, by assisting others with solving their problems I will learn how to deal with, or forget, my own"). He overcomes his own grief or hardships not by self-indulgence or amusement, nor by seeking out new companions or adventure, but by entering into a helping capacity.

Significantly, however, whereas a *Lachesis* is able to derive stimulus, enjoyment, even exhilaration from performing a heavy duty or shouldering an additional burden, *Natrum muriaticum* takes his duties, like his pleasures, seriously—and often sadly. This explains why his aura is so often tinged with sadness: it is the sadness of one who has renounced that most elusive (to him) of all states of being in this life—personal happiness—and who, no longer asking for himself, hopes only to assist in the happiness of others.

Not surprisingly, then, *Natrum muriaticum* possesses prominent reforming impulses. Full of passionate desire to instruct and exhibiting an inordinate concern for the intellectual and spiritual welfare of others, he is convinced that *he* knows how people should think and what they should do to make this world a better one. More than any other type, he takes on (often uninvited) the role of his brother's keeper. Paradoxically, this individual, who so fears being influenced and so adamantly fights guidance, is always trying to guide and influence others. While not wanting to change himself, he is ever anxious to change humanity.

He begins early in life to demonstrate his irrepressible reforming urge by working on the tastes, values, attitudes, even religious beliefs of his nearest and dearest. The aforementioned difficult parental relationship stems in part from his frustration at not being able to reform them. Nor does the reforming instinct abate as *Natrum muriaticum* matures, but is sublimated into reforming others on an expanded social or institutional scale. If asked what offends him most in life, his unhesitating reply will be "unfairness" or "injustice"—and he will generously champion causes to counteract these. Moreover, motivated by an ever-present sense of duty and sustained by feelings of righteousness, he derives a moral satisfaction and fulfillment from his attempts to move the mountains of social injustice that nothing else in his life can supply.

Whatever his field of endeavor, *Natrum muriaticum* frequently displays an intense social consciousness and a powerful humanitarian impulse. But because he tends to champion painful or unpopular causes, his efforts often go unrecognized. While morally right, he may find himself out of step with the world. Either like the early abolitionists, he trumpets his challenge before society is ready to respond or, like Don Quixote, fighting to resurrect the cause of the Knight Errant in Spain, he comes on the scene too late. Yet, even when attacking the existing order, he expects others immediately to salute the controversial flag he has raised. He wants to criticize society freely ("for its own good"), yet expects to be thanked for it. Then he is aggrieved when the thanks are not forthcoming and the world continues along its erroneous path.

Perhaps it is for this reason that despite his good works, *Natrum muriaticum* frequently feels that he has failed in life. The remedy is prescribed for those who are weary from long striving and who are disappointed with the lack of recognition for their unremitting labors—for those who resemble the Prophet Jeremiah crying in the streets of Jerusalem, lamenting his loneliness, his people's failure to heed his admonitions and teachings, and God's failure to reward his righteousness. Certainly, moral approval is a form of approbation the type can never get enough of—and he can be insufferably self-righteous.

Another image that befits him is that of the ugly duckling who takes a long time to come into its own. This is the individual who discovers his true purpose in life only after having gone through much hardship. Only after having learned to attenuate his too high ideals and unrealistic moral expectations, relinquished his uncompromising stance—and above all, come to understand that others must be accorded the same freedom to make their own choices and mistakes in life that he himself insists on—does he become a swan.

Sometimes the "burdened" characteristics described in this chapter will be absent from the *Natrum muriaticum* picture. Either they have been modified by other remedies or the individual has simply been blessed with an unambiguously cheerful disposition (this latter type *does* exist). But in most instances a *Natrum muriaticum* will manifest some of the minor-key features presented here. If he does not now exhibit them, he may have overcome them in the past—or found contentment and a life meaning in some humanitarian work. Alternately, he will admit to a continuing struggle against the festering feelings of misery and sadness ("How can one *not* feel sad," he asks, "with the world so full of reasons to feel so?") or to a tendency to hang on to old injuries with a lobster-claw lock ("I have grown quite attached to them by virtue of their familiarity"). And if a person is actively suffering from long-standing dejection or a severe sorrow or feels out-of-step with the world, is self-condemning, or excessively self-absorbed (as he passes through the lonely transitional stage between separation from his past and discovering a new identity), then it is that the potentized salt can cut through the tangle of introversion, depression, and feelings of unworthiness to enable the sufferer to find that place to stand from which he can, like Archimedes, move the world.

Natrum muriaticum

PRINCIPAL REGIONS AFFECTED

Head Pains of the throbbing, hammering, blinding, migraine variety (often centered around the eyes); **brought on by menses, sun, heat, eyestrain; also by anger, grief, or other strong emotion;** eyes bruised, burning feeling; tired with heavy lids; **worse from reading;** easy lacrymation from laughing, coughing, wind

Heart **Palpitations, especially on lying down;** intermittent heartbeat; tachycardia

Digestion Sleepiness or weariness after eating; perspires on face while eating; **constipation,** sometimes alternating with diarrhea

Urination Involuntary when coughing, sneezing, laughing, walking

Female Vaginal dryness; pain during intercourse; **various complaints before, during, and after menses:** skin eruptions, headache, cramping, low back pains, diarrhea, etc.; **menses** too profuse, **irregular (usually late),** or absent

Skin **Oily, greasy** (especially on face); dry eruption along margin of hairline; **adolescent or adult acne;** fever blisters or cold sores around and canker sores in the mouth; crack in middle of the lower lip; hives break out after exertion or ingestion of some particular food, such as fish or strawberries; crusty eruptions in bends of the limbs and behind the ears

GENERALITIES

Weakness and tiredness felt primarily in neck (must support it with hand); secondarily in lower back, knees and ankles

Sadness exhibited in the lines around eyes and mouth (which, however, can be obliterated by a face-transforming smile)

Fluid retention (a physical counterpart of the inability to let go of unpleasant emotions); general inability to perspire, except when eating

Hay fever diathesis (constitutional predisposition) with much sneezing and nasal discharge of raw egg white consistency

Sleepless from grief or disagreeable emotion (even if long past)

Dreams of robbers, of being chased, of day's difficulties; also, does not remember his dreams

Continued.

Natrum muriaticum—cont'd

MODALITIES (< worse; > better)

Time	< Morning, on awakening; 10:00 AM; sunrise to sunset: alternate days; yearly
	> After sunset (when the burden of surviving the day is over); before breakfast
Temperature	< Heat: of sun, humidity, warm room; intermittent surges of heat; even if chilly cannot tolerate heat
	> Cool air, cold bathing of affected parts; perspiration
Position	> Lying down (except for cough and palpitations); pressure against back
Food/Drink	< Odor of coffee; too much liquid
	> Frequent small meals
	Craves salt, chocolate, crunchy food; sometimes soup and bread; sometimes averse to fish and mollusks
	> Irregular eating; eating only when hungry
Other	< At the seashore (even though is often drawn to the sea)
	> At the seashore
	< Crying; talking of symptoms or troubles; sympathy, consolation
	< Music, which affects him too deeply
	> Laughter
	> When teaching, counseling, helping others

GUIDING MENTAL SYMPTOMS

Sadness, depression, weariness of life; this can make him gloomy, sulky, melancholic

Inability to express emotions or to let go of them; retention of sorrowful or disagreeable thoughts

Ill-effects of grief, anger, fright, resentment, heartbreak, and other strong emotions; history of disappointing or broken relationships

Extreme sensitivity to criticism or reprimand; strong sense of injury: dwells on grievances and humiliations; bears grudges and does not easily forgive or forget

Difficulty crying (except when talking about personal problems)

Reticent, reserved personality; often averse to company (especially wants to be left alone when feeling sad); at the same time feels lonely, isolated when alone; comfortable neither with people nor without

Vicarious suffering

Derives comfort from working for some humanitarian cause

Fears closed spaces (claustrophobia), heights; mental breakdown; people (being injured by them); robbers

Thuja

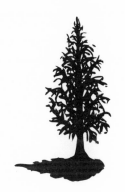

There are more things in heaven and earth, Horatio,
than are dreamt of in your philosophy.

—William Shakespeare, *Hamlet*

The remedy *Thuja occidentalis* is prepared from the twigs and leaves of the *arbor vitae,* a tree belonging to the cypress/cedar family. From ancient times, the cypress has ornamented burial grounds. Its aromatic oil was used in embalming; its decay-resistant wood was used for coffins and, because of its strong fragrance, was burned in sacrificial offerings. Also, according to ancient mythology, this tree was sacred to Pluto, ruler of the underworld and the region of the dead. Thus, in a variety of ways, trees of the cypress family are associated with death. But being a hardy evergreen, capable of surviving in virtually any climate and soil, with its unfading branches holding forth the promise of perpetual existence, the *arbor vitae* is equally associated with immortality. In the following pages we will examine how the concepts of death and eternal life relate to the archetypal picture of *Thuja.*

A prominent physical feature of this constitutional type is the proliferation of cells, manifested most clearly in skin outgrowths and excrescences. These may include moles, corns, fatty tumors, polyps, condylomata, hematomas, and warts of every variety—many of which, in a curious correspondence between nature and man, bear a resemblance to the resinous callosities on the stem and branches of the *arbor vitae.*

On the mental-emotional level, *Thuja* bears a striking resemblance to *Natrum muriaticum.* True, the first impression is of a lighter personality; he does not bear those unmistakable lines of pain or sadness that form around the eyes or mouth—and consequently appears more open and trusting (with its uptilted branches, the *arbor vitae* has a jaunty appearance). This, however, can be deceptive. Like individuals of the salt diathesis, the troubled *Thuja* is apt to view himself as singled out by destiny to be the recipient of Hamlet's "slings and arrows of outrageous fortune." He also evinces the all-too-familiar consequences of repressed emotions: resentment, depression, and difficulty dealing with anger. Additionally, he may shoulder the guilt of the world and tend to absorb, as if they were his own, any spirit-of-the-times injuries or negative emotions currently in circulation. So deeply entrenched are the *Thuja* injuries, personal or vicarious, that sometimes, unlike *Natrum muriaticum,* they cannot—dare not—surface, even in body language.

Also differing from the *Natrum muriaticum* picture is an underlying duality in the *Thuja* nature, which alone is able to account for certain aspects of the personality. For instance, the swiftness with which the individual can switch from amiability to obnoxiousness is astonishing. One moment, he is all openness and loving consideration; the next, secretive, callous, disagreeable. His duality is multifaceted—not limited solely to attitude and social behavior but also encountered in his tastes and preferences. For instance, the individual might harbor a liking for both horror books and movies *and* for refined and even sentimental ones. Or he or she is the athlete who writes esoteric poetry. A committed vegetarian for "spiritual" reasons, he may simultaneously indulge in substance abuse. For friends he chooses both the finest souls among his peers and the most disreputable.

The trunk of the *arbor vitae* is nearly as inflexible as a pillar of salt, and *Thuja,* once again similar to *Natrum muriaticum,* can be characterized by emotional inflexibility and a general inability to go with the flow. More idiosyncratically, and beginning already in infancy, *Thuja* does not respond well to transitions of any nature— either external (a changing environment) or internal (the normal course of growth and development). He suffers greatly from interruptions in whatever he is engrossed, becomes unreasonably distraught over changes in routine, and has rigid notions about the way things are done: when, where, and how. Thus, he may be angered by being asked to walk the dog in the evening instead of his usual afternoon hour or is distressed by a variation of schedule in a shared kitchen; or, developing proprietary claims to communal objects, he can barely endure someone occupying his favorite chair in front of the television. Such minor concerns should be inconsequential compared with larger life issues, as *Thuja* himself realizes perfectly well. Nevertheless, they affect him profoundly: "I find myself fretting over the pettiest, most insignificant matters and upsets in my routine. I can't understand why this should be. Everything is going well with me; yet instead of enjoying my life, some small thing crops up to plague me."

The speaker was touching lightly on a trait that has far-reaching ramifications. Individuals of this constitution find themselves equal to only those situations which are patterned, prepared for, and require of them no adjustments. Such inflexibility and inability to contend with the normal flow of existence reflects deep-seated insecurities that compel *Thuja* to concentrate on unimportant, peripheral matters in an attempt to control the larger, unpredictable ones. Even more: the trait is indicative of fragility and a tenuous mental balance—at times even of an underlying chaos or disorder in the psyche that is on the verge of breaking through. To stave off this last— that is, to propitiate the dark forces threatening to erupt—the individual sets up extra-rigid rules and frameworks within which he can operate in relative security; and then abides by these—with a tenacity!

Last, similar to *Natrum muriaticum, Thuja* often feels ill at ease around people ("Although I may not show it, I feel unwanted and out of place among my peers"; or, "I spend one third of my life dealing with people and the other two thirds recuperating from the experience"). This unease stems from a number of causes, such as a history of neglect, deprivation, or early separation from mother as a result of illness or adoption; or childhood or adult abuse. And such a background can engender in a person more than merely a sense of his own inadequacy and social discomfort. On a deeper level, it engenders feelings of alienation from humanity—of being a stranger in this world.

Natrum muriaticum, we recall, can likewise be a victim of injury, neglect, or an unhappy childhood, and feels himself to be an outsider. No type is more aware of man's intrinsic isolation or is more convinced that he can never be a part of the congenial human scene ("It's always the same old story: never belonging anywhere in this world—always feeling like a second-class citizen"). Nevertheless, although burdened by loneliness and saddened by his inability to establish easy and comfortable relations with other people, he keeps trying to do so. Even while feeling uncomfortable, and at the risk of pain or rejection, he is always endeavoring, by means of a high-minded altruism and by readily sublimating his personal grievance into social and existential concerns, to adjust to the world; his psyche is firmly lodged in this reality. *Thuja*'s estrangement, in contrast, albeit less obvious (because he is socially more adroit), is more radical in nature. His psyche has already begun a protective distancing or disconnecting from this world. Therefore, to properly understand the remedy's uniqueness, one needs to delve beneath a person's conscious mental-emotional levels into the subconscious—and there, in the dark recesses of the psyche, explore the struggles and challenges that constitute the *Thuja* archetype.

Because he has been so profoundly injured in this lifetime, or, as sometimes happens, has been affected by an imagined victimization (this last to be discussed below), a part of *Thuja*'s spirit has withdrawn from this world and unconsciously sought refuge in some other sphere of reality, where it hopes to feel more at ease. In other words, a certain psychic break—a nonintegration between the spirit and mortal frame—has already taken place. Hence the key *Thuja* sensation of feeling "as if his soul were separated from his body." No longer his old self but not yet understanding his new self, he is experiencing the growing pains of transition from an existence entirely in this world to an awareness of other dimensions.

Undergoing the pains of this transition was the man recently returned from a vacation on an island off the Atlantic coast. Contrary to his own expectations (since he usually loved being near the ocean), the vacation had not been a success. He had felt as if the island were haunted, and he was continuously aware of unfriendly spirits beside him, resenting his presence: "It was an eerie and unpleasant sensation that I've never felt there before." Only later did he learn that he had been staying near the alleged burial grounds of an American Indian tribe that had been massacred by white settlers. Another case in point was the *Thuja*-requiring patient who recounted how sometimes at night, just as she was about to fall asleep, she sensed the presence of her departed mother hovering around her. The latter seemed to be trying to tell her daughter something, but it was unclear what, and the experience was unsettling. Later it materialized that the spirit was urging her to see a homoeopath for her rheumatoid arthritis—as, once the daughter complied, the apparitions ceased.

In addition to this type's being extra susceptible during sleep to visitations by departed spirits, the subject matter of many a *Thuja*'s dreams indicates his having ventured over some threshold of this reality into the realm of the dead. He dreams of the dead, of holding lengthy conversations with them, of himself being a denizen of the nether world, or that he is about to become one, and so forth.

Sometimes with *Thuja,* significant changes in consciousness have already started to take place but have not yet been assimilated. In the meantime, the subject resorts to stout denial. Entertaining angels unawares was the man who, although a city resident, had opted to take his entire two-week annual vacation not at a mountain or seaside resort but in New York City (!) so as to attend a conference on Tibetan Buddhism. When asked why he had chosen to do so, he replied airily, "Oh, out of sheer, unadulterated curiosity—nothing more spiritual than that." Yet to subject oneself to a full fortnight of listening to the teachings of Tibetan mystics for gruelingly long hours (when the audience spent most of its time trying to figure out whether the Tibetan interpreters were speaking garbled English or had lapsed into their native tongue) argued for *some* spiritual leanings—none the less valid for being unconscious.

Every person is on a spiritual path of his own, but some individuals, such as clairvoyants, clairaudients, psychics, and mediums, already feel secure in the extrasensory realms. *Phosphorus,* for instance, feels not only at home in these realms, but actually enhanced by extrasensory perceptions. With his highly receptive, impressionable disposition, he eagerly welcomes novel sensations, emotions, and experiences—often consciously cultivating communication with energies from other realities. *Lachesis* lies midway between *Phosphorus* and *Thuja*: he may struggle with the supernatural dimension more than *Phosphorus,* but does not close down to the experience in the way *Thuja* so often initially does. Although somewhat threatened, *Lachesis* feels simultaneously excited and exhilarated by being under the influence of a superhuman force, since this control is often accompanied by surges of heightened creativity.

Thuja appears to be called for during that particular stage in an individual's spiritual development when his particular challenge is to grow more at ease in the new spheres of reality that are opening up to him. Understandably, this stage can be a frightening one. Lost as he is between two worlds, feeling at ease in neither, and psychically disoriented from being subjected to a variety of sensations that take the form of altered or out-of-body experiences, encounters with presences, hearing voices from other planes of reality, and other such brushes with the supernatural—his mind is in a turmoil of bewildering emotions that he can neither comprehend nor control.

In fact, the classic *Thuja* sensations "as if he is made of glass, is brittle, is lighter than air," "that his continuity would be dissolved," or "that his body is separated from his soul" could be viewed as accurately representing his fragile psychic state on the verge of breaking down; while the symptom "feels as if his skull is too tight" or "as if his body were too small for the soul" could reflect the psyche's attempt to break through some barrier or confinement that is preventing *Thuja* from accepting the encroaching new dimensions. Conceivably, also, the type's sensations "as if strangers are approaching and accosting him or that someone is beside or calling him" could well be actual spirit entities that are trying to engage him and make their presence felt. And the "fear of being under superhuman control" may be a legitimate dread felt by this vulnerable and confused individual who, sensing the presence of other energies without understanding them, is living in terror lest he fall unduly under their influence.

It also follows that this individual, who a priori displays a tenuous hold on life and an estrangement from this world (at times to the point of feeling disconnected from this plane of reality), would be the one more easily assailed by past-life experiences—not merely remembered but in some uncontrolled way, relived. This, then, is what was meant earlier by the phrase *imagined victimization.* Imagined, not because it is made up, with no basis or reality to it (that is, the product of a diseased fancy), but because it belongs to another plane of reality than that of this present lifetime.

Finally, that which sets the seal to the psychically vulnerable *Thuja*'s mental-emotional confusion is having no conventional paradigm or frame of reference within which to shape and make sense of his paranormal experiences. Because the human vocabulary is not adequate for describing the phenomena of other planes of reality, the individual's comprehension is not equal to the experienced emotions. And "I don't feel 'inside' my body" or "some weird encounters are taking place in me" or "my soul does not feel integrated with my body" are a few of the more common, hopelessly inadequate ways an individual expresses the spiritual upheavals he is undergoing.

Weighing heavily on the spirits of a homemaker was her recently emerged propensity for hearing voices. Some were minatory and accusing, telling her that she was evil; others were friendly and comforting, telling her she was good. But the combined assault of malignant and benign forces was frightening and confusing, making her "feel double" or "as if divided in two parts" (two other classic *Thuja* symptoms) and wonder if she were possessed. It was only after she received *Thuja* that the woman began to distinguish between the opposing voices and at least partially to comprehend the phenomenon she was experiencing—and consequently to heal. As to her voices: "Oh, I continue to hear them. I suppose they are here to stay. But," she added (with a gracious bow to the inevitable), "I've decided, for the benefit of others as well as myself, to learn how to channel the good and helpful voices."

Not only in this intriguing instance but in a number of similar cases, the potentized *arbor vitae* has proved to be of undeniable value in assisting emotionally scarred patients to brave both the physical and emotional upheavals entailed in the expansion of psychic awareness; also in helping individuals remain grounded during the often unsettling process of spiritual growth.

However, *Thuja*'s growing sensitivity to other levels of consciousness and to the extrasensory dimension need not always be disturbing or fraught with strife. Certain individuals of this type, with their toil and struggles behind them, who are now free to reap the spiritual rewards, experience solely uplifting encounters with spirit entities. For instance, it is often a *Thuja* who will display an anthropomorphism—alleging that nature is permeated with living entities and that he or she senses the presence of living spirits in trees, shrubs, flowers, and even the lowly weeds. But, all too often, individuals of this diathesis have to come to an understanding of psychic phenomena the hard way—that is, through illness or emotional suffering, and the related feelings of alienation from this world.

Finally, it is noteworthy that the *Thuja* symptom "sensation as if his mind were separated from his body" is encountered equally in persons experiencing genuine artistic, psychic, or other forms of inspiration, as in those suffering from spiritual disease and estrangement. For instance, in the performing arts, *Thuja* can be recognized by a transcendent quality—not so much in the sense of excellence or exquisiteness of performance (of which other types are also capable) as in the way a performer brings an unusual, other-worldly quality to his art. The preternatural impression left on the audience is of something so fragile and vulnerable as to be almost too delicate and precariously poised for this world.

Among creative artists, it is Leonardo da Vinci who preeminently evinces the *Thuja* inspirational style. Never feeling entirely at home in this world, suffering from that *Thuja* sense of "foreignness," da Vinci spent much of his adult life wandering from town to town, unable to settle anywhere. When he did settle, he was a recluse, living remote from, and at odds with, society. True, he was born illegitimate; but in the Renaissance, a time when the self-made and self-educated man was respected, illegitimacy was no ineradicable stigma.

This individual, who possibly perceived the world around him with a clearer eye than any man before or since, still revealed, both in his unsettling paintings and in his voluminous notebooks, a soul baffled by an alien environment. Additionally, feelings of alienation from this world compelled da Vinci to learn everything in his own way, starting from scratch, no matter how trivial his object. With his uncompromising rigidity, which worked simultaneously to foster his genius and to obstruct it, he displayed an almost perverse determination to approach even the most familiar phenomena from his own idiosyncratic point of view—always reinventing the wheel. For instance, because he would not accept the time-tested pigments and varnishes of his day, insisting instead on experimenting with his own mixtures of curious ingredients, several of his greatest works (such as *The Last Supper*) deteriorated prematurely. Then, too, in a true *Thuja* saltation from one interest to another, he was forever starting projects of great promise, only to abandon them for intervening ideas. Legend has it that when Pope Leo X commissioned a painting from da Vinci, the artist grew so enthralled with devising a new varnish that eventually the Pope gave up waiting and declared, "Alas! This man will never accomplish anything; for he begins by thinking of the end of the work before the beginning."

This statement proved to be misguided. Although it was true that at a time when artists of da Vinci's stature were turning out paintings by the score, he completed barely a dozen, that which Leo X could not have foreseen was the visionary quality of these few works, every one of which proved to have a major influence on all subsequent European painters. The Pope, however, inadvertently touched on one fundamental aspect of the *Thuja* inspirational mode: an inborn distaste for system, continuity, and finality. An overabundance of ideas (corresponding to the body's earlier mentioned propensity to the overgrowth and overproliferation of cells) impels the type to leap from elaborate preliminary notes, initial sketches, or other forms of preparation, over the necessary intermediary steps of the artistic process, to the gratifying feeling of completion. Unfortunately, the end result might remain haphazard or completed only in thought. It takes a self-discipline out of the ordinary for this type to force himself to slow down—to return to somewhere around stage two or three of his original project—then systematically to take up, one by one, the crucial intermediary steps requisite for completion of his work. Alternately, when *Thuja* does force himself to work systematically, he may go to the other extreme—compulsiveness about minutiae. Either way, whether from a distracting proliferation of ideas interrupting the creative process or from toiling obsessively over trivia and detail, the result can be a particular artist's loss of interest in the project before it sees the light of day.

Last, it is significant that every one of da Vinci's great paintings contains elements of an elusive, brooding, twilight world ("beauty touched with strangeness": Walter Pater) that leaves the viewer feeling baffled and unsettled—in the same way that *Thuja* himself is baffled and unsettled by aspects of other planes of reality crowding in on him. The enigmatic smile of the Mona Lisa (*La Gioconda*) suggests not only the complex inner life, but also conveys a sense of the ambiguous, unexplored regions of the psyche; and the mirage-like landscape in the background has the strangeness of another planet. The artist's love of twisting movement (seen in the poses and love-locks of his figures, his serpentine flowers, and his countless drawings of the movement of wind and turbulent water) can be viewed as mirroring the twistings and convolutions of the *Thuja* psyche. And the disturbing smile and equivocal pose of St. John, in the painting *St. John the Baptist,* in which he points not toward the light or the Christ figure (as he is traditionally represented) but back into impenetrable blackness, hints at the dark unfathomable realms outside our human field of vision. All together, these elements suggest that the artist had peered into realms beyond the empirical—and somehow reflect the hooded, inward-turning nature of a not-entirely-of-this-world *Thuja* genius.

Unlike his famous Renaissance contemporary, Michelangelo, or follower, Raphael, Leonardo da Vinci remains to this day a mysterious figure, with one foot in some strange visionary world—yet who, because he was primarily an artist and not a mystic, held back from venturing further into those shadowy realms, whose haze can only be dispelled by mystical concepts.

These days a *Thuja* picture is recognized with increased frequency in a large variety of disturbances of the emotions and the psyche. Not only is the remedy beneficial for those who are in spiritual crisis, but also for those who have failed to manage their lives successfully or to understand how a satisfying life could be conducted. It also benefits those of insecure ego, who have no order in their mentality, and who grow ever more absorbed in themselves and estranged from others, as they wait for some apology from life, some reparation, some explanation as to why they do not feel at ease in this world. The fact is that *Thuja* illnesses have a way of triggering deeply buried resentments and unacknowledged anger, of bringing to the surface long-suppressed traumas. Regardless of the original source of suffering, the hitherto inchoate and shapeless but smoldering negative emotions, knit up with unarticulated feelings of having been cheated by life, now begins to take on a fixed form. And, like the *Thuja* pattern of overgrowth of undesirable cells, they begin to proliferate and feed on themselves, leaving little space for healthy emotions—and ultimately permitting no entry of light. Then, left without any healing direction, the sufferer finds himself dispirited. Truly, *dis*-spirited. He gets tied up in knots of conflicting emotions (remorse and resentment; touchy pride and abject self-reproach; self-blame and blaming others; loathing of life, yet anger at being left out), which he is in no way capable of disentangling without spiritual guidance. Intellect, instinct, intuition, and good intentions are simply not sufficient.

Certainly, other constitutional types are subject to similar sufferings. Indeed, Samuel Hahnemann consistently claimed that, barring injuries and accidents, all illness is a disease of the spirit ("When a person falls ill it is only [the] spiritual self-sustaining vital force, everywhere present in the organism, that is primarily deranged by the dynamic influence upon it of a morbific agent")* and that his highly diluted medicines addressed the spirit aspect of disease. But it is the idiosyncrasy of the traumatized *Thuja* that without understanding, in archetypal terms, the meaning behind his sufferings, without framing them in a context greater than this life, and especially without some spiritual guidance beyond the self to lead him through the misty regions of the under and middle worlds (as Virgil guided Dante), he cannot truly heal.

Such was the case of a certain physiotherapist with a history of childhood abuse, who suffered from severe headaches, during which time she would experience a complete loss of self-confidence, an aversion to company, an abhorrence of touching others, and a fear of loss of reason. Although a true healer who was helping her clients by means of gentle body adjustments with her remarkable hands, she had no clear comprehension of the powers with which she was working; and a dread of the unknown was restraining her from venturing deeper into the spiritual realm. At one point, she experienced a nervous breakdown. *Thuja* was prescribed, which remedy helped her to overcome a mistrust of and resistance

---

*Organon of Medicine, Section 11. Translated by R.E. Dudgeon. New Delhi, India: B. Jain, Publisher.

to all things metaphysical sufficiently for her to agree to visit a psychic. The latter elucidated (by exploring past lives) the spiritual lesson behind her sufferings and instructed her in techniques for getting in touch with her guiding spirits. "These are teaching me how to welcome even the most trying experiences in life as opportunities for growth—and assisting me to fulfill my role in the Cosmic Plan" (as the *Thuja* woman, availing herself of New Age terminology, put it). Later, she interpreted her now largely cured frontal headaches as the concrete physical expression of her "third [spiritual] eye" attempting to open up, yet being blocked. Thereafter, she required only occasional doses of *Thuja* to keep her "third eye" open and her headaches at bay—and, above all, to help her stabilize while assimilating the changes of enormous magnitude (and what change could be more vast and unsettling than embarking on the uncharted seas of the spirit world?) that she was undergoing in the course of her healing.

In this way, often a breakdown in the old personality, where a person must relinquish certain aspects of his former self (some fears, rigidities, or limiting patterns of behavior) could be viewed as the precursor of a higher integration of body and soul. As with the fabled phoenix rising out of the ashes of its own pyre, the old must die so that the new can live.

Sacrifice or death of the old life and birth of a new one serve as fitting images for *Thuja*'s remarkable healing action on the psyche, as the remedy comes to the aid of those *dis*-spirited patients who, having lost their direction in their current sojourn on earth, must find it in realms beyond the one limited by our five senses. And this picture helps us to appreciate the full significance of this ordinary, often scrub, conifer being endowed with the grandiose name of *arbor vitae*—the "tree of life."

Thuja

PRINCIPAL REGIONS AFFECTED

Head	**Pain as if pierced by a nail** or nagging, stabbing neuralgic pains; dandruff; dry, split hair; tendency to develop styes; agglutinated eyelids at night; chronic nasal catarrh (thick, green); dryness of nasal cavity; painful pressure at root of the nose; tooth decay at the gums
Chest	Stitches in the chest; **asthma** (*Thuja* may benefit when *Arsenicum album* fails to act)
Digestion	Abdominal distention; **much rumbling and gurgling in abdomen; spluttering, gushing, hurried, explosive bowel movements**; constipation—often alternates with diarrhea; rectal pain causes stool to recede
Urination	**Forked stream when urinating;** weak or interrupted stream; sudden, urgent, uncontrolled need to urinate
Male	Inflammation of organs, with cutting pains; urethral discharges, **enlarged prostate**; genital warts
Female	**Left-sided ovarian pain;** ovarian cysts; profuse vaginal discharge (thick greenish); excrescences, polyps, and warts in genital area; menstrual disturbances of all kinds, including headaches and offensive perspiration before onset of menstruation
Skin	Picture of overgrowth and overproliferation of soft tissues: **warts, moles, polyps, skin and fungal growths** of all kinds appear on any part of the body; waxy or oily skin, especially of the face

GENERALITIES

Wandering pains: symptoms move from place to place; more often left-sided

Perspires on uncovered parts of the body; **perspiration smells sour or sweet** (of honey, maple syrup, ketchup); offensive perspiration of feet

Dreams confused, unsettling—suggestive of other planes of reality: of the dead, holding conversations with them; that he is dead or about to die; past-life dreams; visions and apparitions

Ill-effects of vaccination (eczema, asthma, joint pains, etc.; children fail to thrive)

MODALITIES (< worse; > better)

Time	< At night, **especially 3:00 AM** (wakens from an aggravation) and secondarily, 3:00 PM; waxing moon and moonlight; yearly
Temperature	< Cold, damp; heat of bed
	> Cool air, but keeping head warm
Food/Drink	< **Onions,** coffee, tea
	> Garlic (which he likes)
Other	< During ovulation

GUIDING MENTAL SYMPTOMS

Loneliness from feeling detached from this world (a "stranger in his own land")

Sadness from feelings of guilt, isolation, and low self-esteem (deeply affected by music)

Feelings of fragility; as if soul were separated from the body

Sensitive, compassionate nature; but also **rigid mentality** and fixed ideas

Altered-body or out-of-body experiences; supernatural or paranormal experiences

Sensation as if someone were beside him; of his being in the hands of a superior power; as if something were alive in his body

Fear of heights, of falling; of losing his reason; of falling under superhuman control; **of transitions;** anxiety over trifling changes

Conclusion

From the observations made in these pages comes the recognition that homoeopathic medicines achieve their profound effects in strengthening the life force and restoring harmony and balance to the human organism precisely because they direct themselves to the unconscious level of a patient's psyche and address his underlying archetypal picture.

Few people, however, are pure types. Although an individual may display characteristics of predominantly one remedy and can thus be considered that particular constitutional type, seldom will a remedy cover his totality of symptoms for all time. Humans are complex and many-layered—and always responding to their environment. The stream of life is sometimes broad and calm, sometimes narrow and turbulent, constantly affected by the tributaries feeding into it. A child's strong manifestation of a *Calcarea carbonica* symptomatology changes as he grows older—or the world would be peopled almost exclusively with *Calcarea carbonica* adults. The *Sepia* housewife was not necessarily always so—and will shed the *Sepia* picture when her children are grown and gone. A patient detoxifying from too much "high living" will require *Nux vomica* for a period of time—perhaps for the only time in his life. Persons needing *Natrum muriaticum* are often in a transitional stage of their emotional and intellectual development and, once they emerge, may eventually manifest characteristics of another constitutional type. The conflicts and doubts typical of *Lachesis* often surface in women in middle age, whereas the *Sulphur* religious and existential anxieties might appear in men during their later years. The stream flows on, expanding or narrowing, becoming deeper or shallower. And with the changing circumstances of life, the personality picture changes, taking on attributes of one remedy or another.

In other words, the homeopathic typology could be viewed as illustrating the different *stages* of a person's growth and development. And a given remedy, by acting on the subconscious and spiritual levels, as well as on the conscious mental-emotional and physical ones, can help the individual to resolve the archetypal conflicts and challenges that he is forever confronting in his passage through life.

Suggested Readings

The following books will aid the reader in further exploration of homoeopathy; all are currently in print.

Boericke, William. *Materia Medica With Repertory.* New Delhi: B. Jain, Publishers (n.d.).

> An indispensable reference work and learning tool for the serious student—the "homoeopathic bible." This text provides the principal bibliographical material for the charts developed in *Nature and Human Personality.* Other editions are also available.

Coulter, Catherine R. *Portraits of Homeopathic Medicines: Psychophysical Analyses of Selected Constitutional Types,* Volumes 1-3. St. Louis: Quality Medical Publishing, 1998.

> These three volumes, published in 1985, 1988, and 1998, explore in greater depth and variety the homoeopathic constitutional types. The archetypal "sketches" in *Nature and Human Personality* are abridged versions of some of the portraits found in this larger work. Extensive bibliographical acknowledgments and specific references can be found in them.

Hahnemann, Samuel. *Organon of the Medical Art.* Edited and annotated by Wenda Brewster O'Reilly, based on a translation by Steven Decker. Redmond, Washington: Birdcage Books, 1996.

> The basic treatise on the homoeopathic philosophy, by the founder of homoeopathy. There are several different translations of this work, any one of which is excellent.

Kent, James Tyler. *Repertory of the Homoeopathic Materia Medica.* New Delhi: B. Jain, Publishers (n.d.).

> The classic text for prescribing, suited to the more advanced student. There are a number of versions of this work.

Panos, Maesimund B., and Heimlich, Jane. *Homoeopathic Medicine at Home*. Los Angeles: JB Tarcher, 1980.

> An excellent introductory book for the beginner, explaining the homoeopathic philosophy and method, and giving indications for prescribing for acute conditions. This is one of a number of books available on this subject.

Index